Acknowledgments

The Foundations for Caregiving course and materials were developed and produced through a joint effort of the American Red Cross and the Mosby Publishing Company. The effort has been a labor of love by individuals who care deeply about the kind of care they will receive from nurse assistants when they and their loved ones are ill. Hopefully, all will be trained through the American Red Cross Foundations for Caregiving Program.

Members of the development team at the American Red Cross who designed and wrote these materials included: Cindy Green, M.P.H., and Carolyn Branson, R.N., B.S.N., Project Leaders; Paula Virgin, R.N., B.S.N., Content Specialist/Writer; Linda Wolfe Keister, Managing Editor; Jill Tunick Assistant Editor; Carol Hunter-Geboy, Ph.D., Instructional Design Consultant; Sharon Dorfman, Education and Evaluation Consultant; Peggy Casey, R.N., Margaret Draganac, R.N., M.P.H., Kathleen Masucci, R.N., Judy Peterson, R.N., B.S.N., Rosemary A. Sullivan, R.N., M.Ed.; and Angie S. Turner, R.N., B.S.N., Red Cross Staff Writers; Margaret Callanan, R.N., Deborah Makie Canavan, R.N., B.S.N., Richard S. Ferri, R.N., Ph.D., CRNI, Alexandra Greeley, Pat Hyland, R.N., Rosa Kasper, Jeff Malter, Lisa Malter, Sharon Romm, Joan Timberlake, Barbara E. Tucker, B.S.N., M.P.H., and Ruth G. Wiskind, R.N., M.N., External Writers.

The following individuals provided additional assistance: Esther Silva, R.N., B.S., M.A., Amy Coats, M.Ed., and Meg A. Riley, Artwork coordinators; Melissa Andrews, copy editor; Alison Hilton, Analyst; Venus Ray, Project Assistan/Proofreader; Cynthia Yockey, Desktop Publisher; Lou Ellen Bell, R.N., B.S.N., M.N., Claudette Clunan, R.N., B.S.N., M.A., Fay Flowers, R.N., M.Ed., Genevieve Gipson, R.N., M.Ed., Katherine Graves, R.N., Carole K. Kauffman, R.N., M.P.H., Diane H. Munro, R.N., M.B.A., and Karne J. Peterson, Ph.D., Internal Reviewers; Lynda Ramsey Bradshaw, L.P.N., B.S., and Sandy Johnson, R.N., Technical Reviewers/Assistant Artwork Coordinators; Charles Pierpont, Assistant Source Photographer and Desktop Publisher; and Tara Theodore, Secretary.

The Mosby production team included: David T. Culverwell, Publisher; Richard A. Weimer, Executive Editor; Mary Beth Ryan Warthen and Julie Scardiglia, Developmental Editors; Gayle May Morris, Project Manager; Mary Cusick Drone, Senior Production Editor; Joan Herron, Desktop Publisher; Kay Kramer, Director, Art and Design; and Betty Schulz and John Rokusek, designers.

Special thanks to Vincent Knaus and Jeannette Ortiz-Osorio, Photographers; and Joe Chovan, Kurt Peterson, Patti Restle, Lisa Petkun, and Michael Cooley, illustrators.

These materials could not have been completed without the generous assistance in time, materials, and manpower of the Fairfax Nursing Center, Fairfax, Virginia; Grant Park Nursing Center, Washington, D.C.,; the National Capital Chapter of the American Red Cross; Peoples Drug, Bailey's Crossroads, Virginia; and Thomas Silva.

The Development Team of Health Care Training extends sincere appreciation to our American National Red Cross paid and volunteer staff for their assistance in completing these materials.

American Red Cross
Skills for Caregiving

American Red Cross Skills for Caregiving

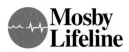

Mosby
Lifeline

St. Louis Baltimore Boston Chicago London Madrid Philadelphia Sydney Toronto

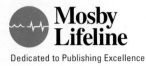

Mosby Lifeline
Dedicated to Publishing Excellence

Printed in the United States of America
Composition by Mosby Electronic Production, St. Louis
Printing/binding by Color Art, Inc.

Mosby-Year Book, Inc.
11830 Westline Industrial Drive
St. Louis, Missouri 63146

Library of Congress Cataloging in Publication Data

Skills for caregiving / American Red Cross.
      p.   cm.
  To be used with: Foundation for caregiving / American Red Cross.
c1993.
  ISBN 0-8016-6514-0
  1. Nurses' aids. 2. Care of the sick--Problems, exercises, etc.
I. American Red Cross. II. Foundations for caregiving.
  [DNLM: 1. Caregivers--education--programmed instruction. 2. Home
Care Services--programmed instruction. 3. Home Nursing--education-
-programmed. 4. Nurse's Aides--education--programmed instruction.
WY 18 S6285 1993]
RT84.F68 1993 Suppl.
610.73 ' 076--dc20
DNLM/DLC
for Library of Congress

93   94   95   96   97   /   9   8   7   6   5   4   3   2   1

Introduction

As a nurse assistant, you perform many important skills every day. You must perform these skills accurately, professionally, and with care for the needs and wishes of the patient, resident, or client. This workbook will guide you as you learn step by step how to perform 74 skills. It is intended to be used with the **Foundations for Caregiving** textbook as part of the American Red Cross Foundations for Caregiving course. The textbook emphasizes six principles of care: safety, infection control, privacy, dignity, independence, and communication.

Most skills are presented in the same brief, easy-to-follow form. Preparation and completion steps are nearly the same for each skill; thus they are called standards. Look at *Skill 6: Taking and Recording a Person's Oral Temperature with a Glass Thermometer* on page 19 to see how a typical skill is organized.

Every skill begins with **Precautions.** This section provides you with a list of things you should think about before you start the skill. Precautions are often based on the principle of safety.

In most skills, a section called **Preparation** follows the precautions. Preparation **standards** are set up in a shortened form, which will be described later in this section. They are concerned mainly with practicing infection control, providing privacy, promoting dignity and independence, and communicating.

The **Procedure** section describes the steps you take that are specific to a particular skill. During the American Red Cross training course, you must learn to do each skill exactly as it is described. However, when you begin to work, your employer may require you to perform the skill somewhat differently. Discuss any differences with your supervising nurse.

The last section of each skill contains **Completion standards**, which are concerned mainly with leaving the person safe and comfortable. You will notice that the layout of the preparation and completion sections is similar. Completion standards are described in greater detail later in this section.

Preparation Standards

The preparation section is divided into the following: 10 boxes that contain a shortened form of each preparation task (called buttons because they resemble the layout of the buttons of some telephones), an Additional Information box, and a Notes box for you to jot down any special points you want to remember.

The borders of the buttons will vary with every skill. Buttons with solid borders and those with double borders contain tasks that you will perform for the skill. If a button has a double border, it means that you will need more information about the task. You will find this information in the shaded Additional Information box. If a button has a dashed border, it means that you do not have to do that step for the skill.

Remember to refer to your textbook for more information about each of the skills. Good luck as you prepare for a most rewarding and vital career.

Look at the sample preparation page on page ii as you read the description of each button.

Skill 6: Taking and Recording a Person's Oral Temperature with a Glass Thermometer

Precautions

- Never take an oral temperature if the person—

    Has had recent mouth surgery or has mouth disease.

    Is getting oxygen.

    Is short of breath or is having trouble breathing.

    Is confused or unconscious.

    Is paralyzed on one side of his body or face.

    Is breathing through his mouth instead of his nose.

    Has a tube in his nose.

    Is under 5 years of age.

- Use only a glass thermometer that is in perfect condition, not one that is chipped, cracked, or broken.

Preparation

1. Gather supplies.
- Oral thermometer (if the person does not have one at his bedside)
- Thermometer sheath (optional)
- Watch with a second hand
- Cotton balls and tissues
- Plastic trash bag
- Paper towels
- Pencil and paper to write down the temperature ☐ ☐

Additional Information

5. If the person has eaten, smoked, or had anything to drink in the past 15 minutes, tell him that you will be back in 15 minutes to take his temperature. Ask him not to eat, smoke, or drink until you return.

8. Gather the person's own thermometer and holder, if they are kept at his bedside.

- Take the thermometer to the sink and clean it, unless you are bringing a clean one with you to the person's room. Shake down the thermometer.

2. Focus ☐ ☐

3. Knock and wait ☐ ☐

4. Introduce and identify ☐ ☐

5. Explain ☐ ☐

6. Place supplies ☐ ☐

7. Wash hands ☐ ☐

8. Gather and prepare ☐ ☐

9. Adjust bed ☐ ☐

10. Provide privacy ☐ ☐

Notes:

Button 1. Gather supplies and equipment not stored in the person's room to save time. Carefully think through the procedure before you perform it in order to provide safe and efficient care. Incidents may occur if you leave a person unattended while you go for something you have forgotten. In this text it is necessary to make some assumptions about where supplies are kept. Therefore, you may need to adapt the procedure to your own work situation.

Button 2. Focus on the person who will receive your care as you gather supplies and think about the task to be done.

You may recall that the person has been unhappy about something. Focus on how you might help her feel better. If you let the person know that you remember things from a previous conversation, she will know that you see her as an individual.

Think about the person's ability to participate in the care. For example, if you know that a person is weak and unable to stand for more than a few seconds, you can plan to have a co-worker help you move her into a chair and make arrangements for help before you actually need it.

Button 3. Knock on the door before entering the person's room **and wait** a moment for permission to enter. If the door is partially or completely opened, you still knock and ask permission to enter, or say, "Excuse me, may I ...?" In this way, you show respect for the person's dignity and privacy.

If the person does not respond, knock a little louder and call her name. If she still does not respond, go into the room, calling her name. In a situation in which the person does not respond to a knock on the door, you must make a choice between respecting the person's privacy and ensuring her safety. In every situation, the safety of the person in your care is your most important responsibility.

Button 4. Introduce yourself to the person **and identify** her by calling her name and checking her name band. If the person is at home, she probably won't be wearing a name band, but you still must verify that you have the right person.

Introducing yourself is common courtesy and promotes the dignity of the person. When you introduce yourself, ask the person how she would like to be addressed and tell her what to call you. Always call a person by her last name and title, such as Mrs. Ryan, unless she tells you that she prefers to be called by another name as the character Josie in the textbook does. If you bring a co-worker to assist you, you should introduce him or her to the person in your care.

Button 5. Explain what you would like to do, such as take vital signs or help with her bath. Ask her what parts of the skill she can do for herself. By involving the person in her care, you promote her independence and gain her cooperation. If you explain a procedure before you begin, you also reduce the possibility of anxiety and confusion.

Button 6. Place the **supplies** on a clean surface, such as an overbed table, or a nightstand. The floor is not considered a clean surface.

Button 7. Wash your **hands.** Handwashing is the single most effective way to reduce the spread of infection. *You should wash your hands as soon as possible after entering the person's room and before touching the person or her personal things.* This reduces the number of new germs you bring from another area into the person's room.

The location of sinks varies from place to place, with some located inside and some outside the room or the privacy curtain. You must know your location and wash your hands so that they are clean before performing a procedure. If you do another task that may have soiled your hands before performing the intended procedure, wash them again. Remember to use a paper towel to turn the faucet on and off, because the faucet handles may transmit germs.

Button 8. Gather the person's own things **and prepare** the supplies and equipment needed. What is available at the person's bedside varies from situation to situation. You must be familiar with your location and adapt the instructions to your particular circumstances. Make sure that the equipment is ready for use. For example, if you are assisting with mouth care, prepare the mouthwash solution. This is also the time to prepare a plastic trash bag or laundry bag if you need it for the procedure and to place it in an appropriate and accessible place.

Button 9. Adjust the **bed** to a working height. This height will vary, depending on the task you have to perform and your safety and comfort needs and those for whom you provide care. For example, when you give a bed bath, the bed should be at about the height of your waist. Or, if you are moving someone up in bed, the height would be lower to promote proper body mechanics.

Note: If the bed does not raise or lower, you must be especially careful to maintain proper body mechanics so that you do not injure your back. If the bed has a hand crank to raise and lower it, use a paper towel to turn the crank to prevent contaminating your hands.

Button 10. Provide privacy in a hospital or nursing home by pulling the bedside curtain all the way around the bed. If you are in a home, make sure the door to the room is closed. This gives the person privacy and dignity while you perform the procedure.

Completion Standards

The completion section follows the procedure steps. It also contains buttons and an Additional Information box that describe the activities you must do when you have completed the procedure. It concludes with lines for you and your instructor to sign and date when you have successfully completed a skill.

As in the Preparation section, each button contains two check-off boxes to be used by your instructor. Look at the sample conclusion page as you read the description of each button.

Completion

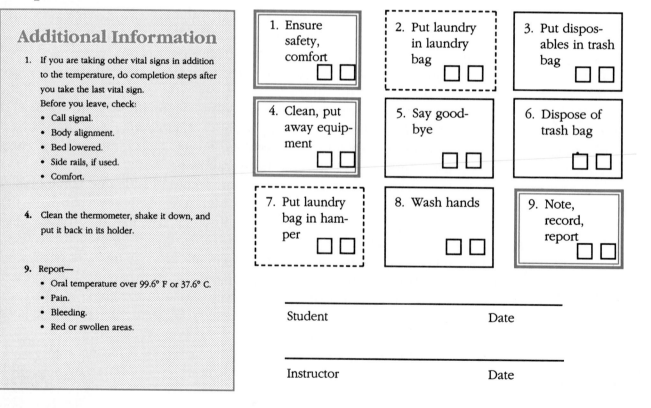

Additional Information

1. If you are taking other vital signs in addition to the temperature, do completion steps after you take the last vital sign.
   Before you leave, check:
   • Call signal.
   • Body alignment.
   • Bed lowered.
   • Side rails, if used.
   • Comfort.

4. Clean the thermometer, shake it down, and put it back in its holder.

9. Report—
   • Oral temperature over 99.6° F or 37.6° C.
   • Pain.
   • Bleeding.
   • Red or swollen areas.

1. Ensure safety, comfort

2. Put laundry in laundry bag

3. Put disposables in trash bag

4. Clean, put away equipment

5. Say good-bye

6. Dispose of trash bag

7. Put laundry bag in hamper

8. Wash hands

9. Note, record, report

Student _____ Date _____

Instructor _____ Date _____

Button 1. Ensure the person's **safety** and **comfort.** Make sure the person's body is in proper alignment. Alignment refers to the position of the person's body in a bed or chair. Proper alignment means that she is comfortable and not twisting or straining any part of her body. (You will read more about good body alignment in Chapter 9, Positioning and Transferring People.) Before leaving the person's room, make sure that she is not only comfortable, but safe.

Ensuring a person's safety includes making sure that the *call signal* is within reach; the *side rails* are up, if necessary; personal articles are within reach; and lighting is adequate. You also may need to return the bed to its *lowest position* to finish the procedure with the person.

Button 2. Put wet or soiled **laundry in** a **laundry bag.** Roll wet laundry so that the wet portions are on the inside and put it in a leakproof bag. Bag laundry where it is used to minimize handling and to control the spread of infection.

Button 3. Put all **disposable(s)** items **in** the plastic **trash bag.**

Button 4. Clean and **put away** all **equipment.** Put on clean disposable gloves if you might come into contact with blood or other potentially hazardous body fluids. Clean the nightstand and overbed table. (If you used gloves, dispose of them in the plastic trash bag.) Cleaning not only controls infection, but it makes the person's environment more pleasant.

Button 5. Say good-bye before leaving.

Button 6. Dispose of the plastic **trash bag** in the dirty utility room or, if you are in a home, in a covered trash container.

Button 7. Put the **laundry bag in** the laundry **hamper.**

Button 8. Wash your **hands.**

Button 9. Note, record, report. Use your notes to record the procedure in the appropriate place. Report any unusual findings to your supervising nurse so that you can discuss the person's care and report any changes in her condition. Ask the person if she wants the privacy curtain or door opened or closed, and respect her wishes.

You will notice two small boxes inside each of the buttons and beside each step of the procedure. These are call check-off boxes and will be used by your instructor. When you believe you can perform the skill without coaching, you will demonstrate the skill for your instructor. The instructor will then place a check in the first box as you do each step. Should you have difficulty and need to demonstrate the skill another time, the instructor will check the second box.

Contents

Skill 1: First Aid for Choking (Airway Obstruction)

Precautions

- If the person can cough forcefully, talk, and breathe, even if it is a wheeze, do not interfere with his attempt to cough up the object.
- If coughing persists, call EMS for help.
- If the person has partial airway obstruction with poor air exchange should be dealt with as if it were complete airway obstruction.

Procedure

Option 1: First Aid for a Conscious Choking Adult or Child Over Age 1: Abdominal Thrusts

1. If the person is alert and oriented, *determine if he is choking.*
   - Ask him "Are you choking?"
   - If he cannot cough, speak, or breathe; shout, "HELP!" A person who is not alert may not understand the question, "Are you choking?" However, you can assess airway obstruction by recognizing coughing, voice sounds, and breathing. ☐ ☐

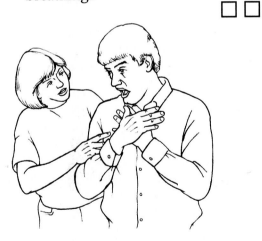

2. *Phone EMS for help.* Tell someone nearby to call for an ambulance or get the supervising nurse who will call EMS. ☐ ☐

Say "Airway is obstructed—Call local EMS number or operator."

3. *Perform abdominal thrusts* (Heimlich maneuver).
   - Stand behind the person and wrap your arms around his waist.
   - Make a fist with one hand. Place the thumb side of your fist against the middle of the person's abdomen, just *above the navel and well below the lower tip of the breastbone.* ☐ ☐

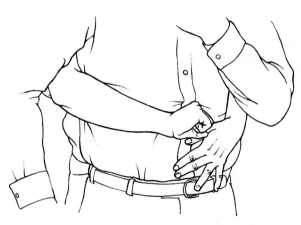

   - Grasp your fist with your other hand.

- Keeping elbows out from the person, press your fist into his abdomen with a *quick upward thrust.* Do not direct the thrust to the right or to the left. Each thrust should be a separate and distinct attempt to dislodge the object that is obstructing his airway.

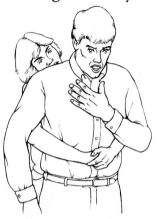

- Repeat thrusts until the obstruction is cleared or the person becomes unconscious.
- If the person coughs up the object or starts to breathe or cough, continue to watch him to make sure he is breathing again. Even though he may be breathing well, remember that he may have other problems that may require a doctor's attention. It is best that the person be examined by more advanced medical personnel.

Option 2: First Aid for a Conscious Choking Adult: Chest Thrusts

To perform chest thrusts on a conscious person who is obese or pregnant, do the following procedure with the person either standing or sitting:

1. Stand behind the person and place your arms under the armpits and around the chest. □ □

2. Place thumb side of your fist on the middle of the breastbone. □ □

3. Grasp your fist with your other hand. □ □

4. Give thrusts against her chest until the obstruction is cleared or the person loses consciousness. □ □

Note: If the object on which the person is choking is not quickly coughed up by your attempts to help, the person may become unconscious. You will probably have some warning that this is about to happen. The person may begin to fall forward or back toward you. Should this occur, lower her to the floor and once more call for help. Stay with the person until help arrives.

The steps to follow for an unconscious person are not part of this course. However, you may take an American Red Cross First Aid or Cardiopulmonary Resuscitation (CPR) Course to learn these steps.

_____

Student   Date

_____

Instructor   Date

2

Skill 2: Handwashing

Precautions

- Do not wear rings to work, except for a simple wedding band.

Why? The tiny spaces in jewelry provide excellent breeding places for germs, which may spread from one person to another.

Procedure

1. Get three paper towels. ☐ ☐

2. Remove your watch, or push it up on your forearm, and roll up your sleeves. ☐ ☐

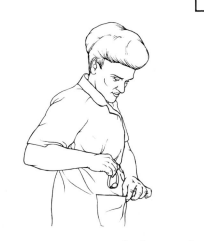

Why? Handwashing includes washing the wrists.

Note: If you cannot wear your watch above your wrist, keep it in your pocket or pin it to your uniform.

3. Turn on the water and adjust the temperature until it is comfortably warm. ☐ ☐

Note: If the water faucet is the kind you must twist on with your hand, use a clean paper towel to turn it on.

Why? Faucet handles are considered dirty and may spread germs.

4. Put your hands under the running water to wet your hands and wrists. ☐ ☐

5. Apply antimicrobial soap from the dispenser. Keep your hands and wrists below the level of your elbows from this point on in the handwashing procedure. ☐ ☐

Why? When you hold your hands and wrists in this position, water runs from the clean area of your forearms to the dirty area of your fingers.

Note: If you must use bar soap, rinse the soap before and after using it.

6. Rub your hands together vigorously to work up a lather. ☐ ☐

Why? Briskly rubbing your hands together helps increase the lather and loosen and remove dirt and germs.

7. Wash for at least 10 seconds, paying particular attention to—
 • The wrists (grasp and circle with your other hand). ☐ ☐

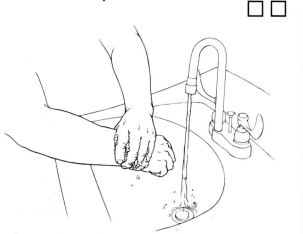

 • The palms and backs of your hands.
 • The area between each finger.

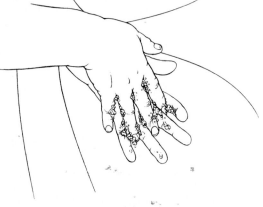

 • The nails (rub against the palms of your hands).

Why? Doing this ensures that you clean all areas thoroughly.

Note: If your hands are contaminated with any body fluids, wash them for longer than 10 seconds.

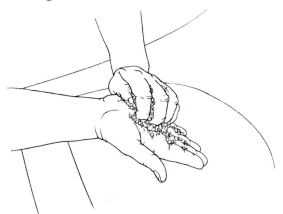

8. Rinse your hands and wrists under the running water. ☐ ☐

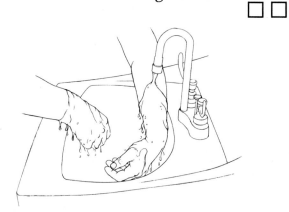

9. Using a clean paper towel, dry your hands thoroughly, beginning at the fingertips and moving back toward the elbow. ☐ ☐

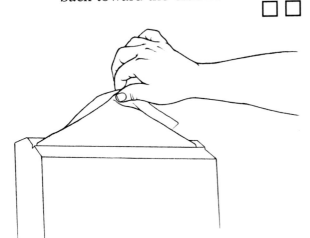

Why? Drying your hands thoroughly keeps them from becoming chapped.

10. Use a clean paper towel to turn off the faucets. ☐ ☐

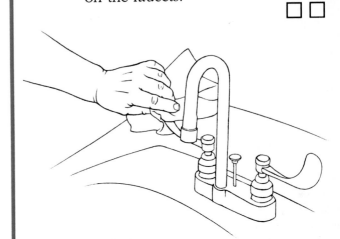

Why? By touching the faucet handles indirectly, you prevent your clean hands from getting contaminated by the dirty handles.

11. Throw away the paper towels in a plastic trash bag. ☐ ☐

Additional Information

Note: If water conservation is a concern, you may use a fresh paper towel to turn off the water after you first wet your hands and then use another paper towel to turn on the water when you are ready to rinse them. Use a fresh paper towel each time you touch the faucet.

_____

Student   Date

_____

Instructor   Date

Skill 3: Putting On and Taking Off Protective Clothing

Precautions

- Usually, put on the protective clothing outside the person's room.
- Change the mask when it becomes moist or after you have been wearing it for 20 minutes.
- Use only gloves that are in perfect condition. If you choose gloves that are cracked, discolored, punctured, or torn, discard them and choose another pair.
- Usually, take off the gloves, mask, and gown in the person's room and discard them as contaminated waste.

Preparation

1. Gather supplies
   - Gown
   - Mask
   - Gloves
   - Plastic trash bag
   - Label or red contamination bag, ☐ ☐ if needed

Additional Information

- Put on the gown, then the mask, then the gloves.

- Take off the gloves, then the mask, then the gown.

2. Focus ☐ ☐

3. Knock and wait ☐ ☐

4. Introduce and identify ☐ ☐

5. Explain ☐ ☐

6. Place supplies ☐ ☐

7. Wash hands ☐ ☐

8. Gather and prepare ☐ ☐

9. Adjust bed ☐ ☐

10. Provide privacy ☐ ☐

Notes:

Procedure

The six tasks for putting on and taking off protective clothing are as follows:

1. Putting on a gown
2. Putting on a mask
3. Putting on disposable gloves
4. Taking off disposable gloves
5. Taking off a mask
6. Taking off a gown

Task 1: Putting On a Gown

1. Slide your arms through the arm-holes, so the opening of the gown is in the back. ☐ ☐

2. Fasten the ties at the back of your neck and at your waist so that the gown covers all of your clothing. ☐ ☐

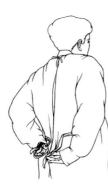

Task 2: Putting On a Mask

1. Put the mask over your mouth and nose and bend the nose wire. ☐ ☐

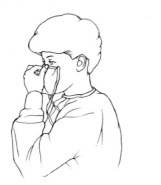

2. Tie the top strings behind your head and then tie the bottom strings. If the mask has elastic ear loops, fit them securely over each ear. ☐ ☐

3. Adjust the mask for comfort. ☐ ☐

Task 3: Putting On Disposable Gloves

1. Inspect both gloves carefully, making sure neither one has any holes. ☐ ☐

2. Put the gloves on carefully, so that they don't tear. Pull the gloves up over the gown cuffs. ☐ ☐

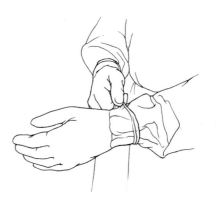

Task 4: Taking Off Disposable Gloves

1. Using your fingers on your gloved left hand, make a cuff on the glove on your right hand, grasp the cuff on the palm side, and pull the glove down toward the fingers of your right hand. Remove the glove only partway. ☐ ☐

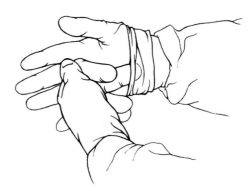

Note: While cuffing the glove, touch only the outside of the glove with the gloved left hand.

Why? The inside of the glove is clean.

2. Using your fingers on your right hand, take off the glove on your left hand by pulling it inside out and rolling it into a ball, without touching your bare left hand. ☐ ☐

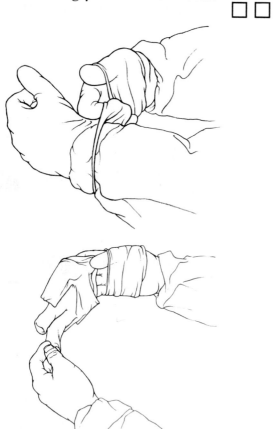

3. Continue to hold the left-hand glove that you have removed in your right hand. ☐ ☐

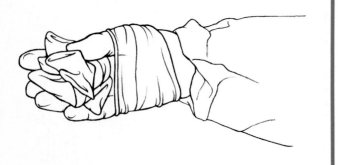

4. With your bare left hand, grasp the glove on your right hand, touching only the clean inside of the glove. ☐ ☐

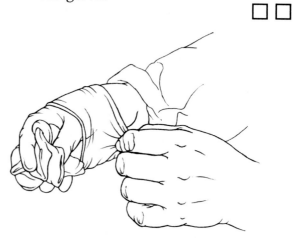

5. Remove the right-hand glove by pulling it down so that the left-hand glove you removed is now inside the right-hand glove. ☐ ☐

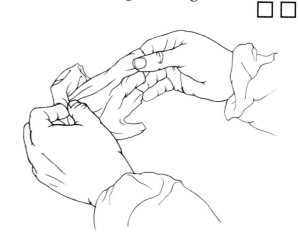

☐ ☐

6. Throw away the gloves in a plastic trash bag or covered trash container. ☐ ☐

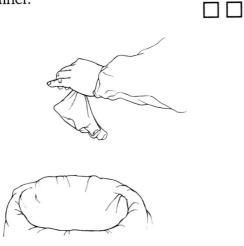

7. Wash your hands now if you are not wearing any other protective gear (mask, gown). Otherwise continue taking off your mask and then your gown and then wash your hands.

Task 5: Taking Off a Mask

1. Untie the bottom strings and then the top strings, or pull the elastic loop from around one ear and then the other. ☐ ☐

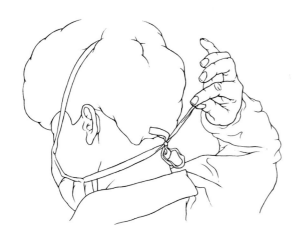

2. Hold the mask by the strings and throw it away in a plastic bag or a covered trash container. ☐ ☐

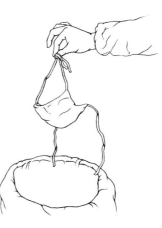

Task 6: Taking Off a Gown

1. Untie the gown in the back. ☐ ☐

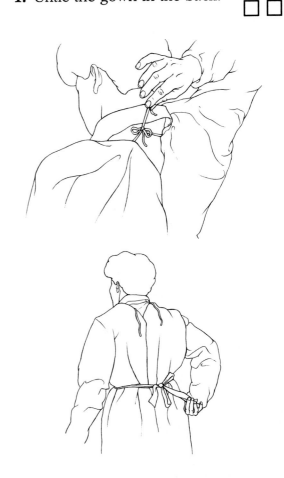

2. Pull off one gown sleeve by slipping your fingers under the cuff and pulling the sleeve just over your fingertips. ☐ ☐

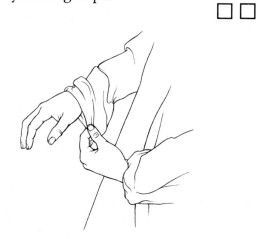

Note: Remember that the end of the sleeve is clean because it was covered by the glove.

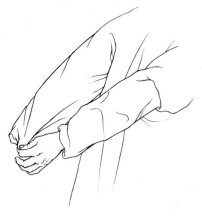

3. Grasp the other sleeve with the covered hand and pull it off. ☐ ☐

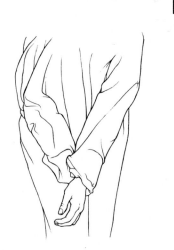

4. Continue holding that sleeve in your covered hand. Grasp the inside of the first shoulder of the gown with your uncovered hand and pull the gown off the shoulder. Continue to bring the gown forward and turn it inside out as you pull it over your covered hand. ☐ ☐

5. Fold the outer, contaminated surface inward and roll up the gown. ☐ ☐

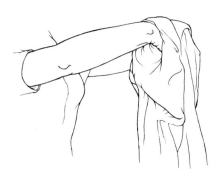

6. Throw the gown in the laundry hamper, plastic trash bag, or covered trash container.

7. Wash your hands. ☐ ☐

Completion

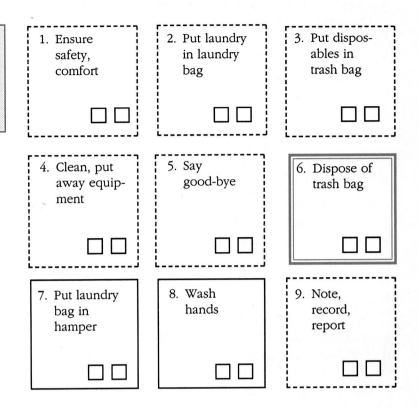

1. Ensure safety, comfort ☐ ☐

2. Put laundry in laundry bag ☐ ☐

3. Put disposables in trash bag ☐ ☐

4. Clean, put away equipment ☐ ☐

5. Say good-bye ☐ ☐

6. Dispose of trash bag ☐ ☐

7. Put laundry bag in hamper ☐ ☐

8. Wash hands ☐ ☐

9. Note, record, report ☐ ☐

_____

Student   Date

_____

Instructor   Date

Skill 4: Handling a Plastic Trash Bag

Precautions

- When closing a dirty trash bag, touch only the outside of the bag, because the inside of the bag is contaminated.

Preparation

1. Gather supplies
   - Plastic trash bag(s) □ □

Additional Information

1. When double bagging will be required, arrange for a co-worker to assist you at a certain time.

2. Focus □ □

3. Knock and wait □ □

4. Introduce and identify □ □

5. Explain □ □

6. Place supplies □ □

7. Wash hands □ □

8. Gather and prepare □ □

9. Adjust bed □ □

10. Provide privacy □ □

Notes:

Procedure

The three tasks for handling a plastic trash bag are as follows:

1. Opening a plastic trash bag

2. Closing a used plastic trash bag

3. Double bagging contaminated trash or laundry

Task 1: Opening a Plastic Trash Bag

1. Open the plastic trash bag and make a cuff around the opened edge. ☐ ☐

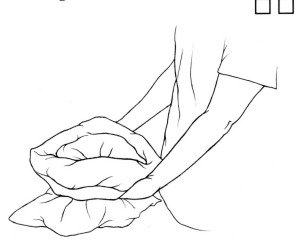

2. Put the opened bag on a clean surface within easy reach of your work area. ☐ ☐

Task 2: Closing a Used Plastic Trash Bag

1. Put your fingers under the cuffed edge of the used plastic trash bag. ☐ ☐

2. Pull the cuffed edges together and close the bag. ☐ ☐

Note: Be sure to touch only the outside of the used bag, because the inside is contaminated.

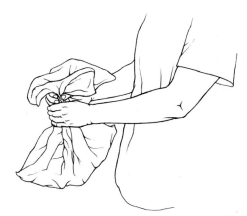

Task 3: Double Bagging a Bag that is Contaminated with Body Fluids

1. Arrange with a co-worker to assist you at a certain time. ☐ ☐

2. Remove the bag from the trash or laundry container inside the isolation room, close it, and carry it to the door of the isolation room. ☐ ☐

3. Have your co-worker prepare a clean bag by folding down a cuff at the top of the clean bag. Have your co-worker hold the clean bag under the cuff and stand by the doorway. ☐ ☐

4. Put the bag with contaminated items into the clean bag that your co-worker is holding under the cuff. ☐ ☐

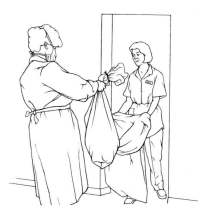

5. Have your co-worker close the outside bag by raising the cuffed area and sealing it shut. ☐ ☐

13

Completion

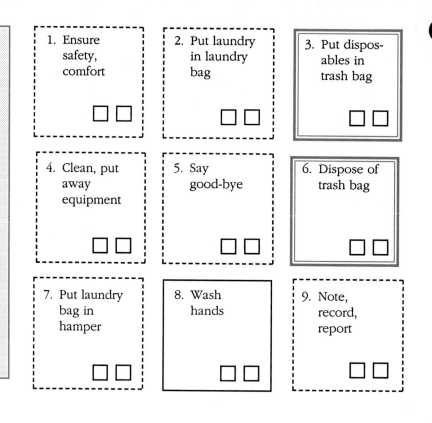

1. Ensure safety, comfort ☐ ☐

2. Put laundry in laundry bag ☐ ☐

3. Put disposables in trash bag ☐ ☐

4. Clean, put away equipment ☐ ☐

5. Say good-bye ☐ ☐

6. Dispose of trash bag ☐ ☐

7. Put laundry bag in hamper ☐ ☐

8. Wash hands ☐ ☐

9. Note, record, report ☐ ☐

Student _____ Date

Instructor _____ Date

14

Skill 5: Reading, Cleaning, and Shaking Down a Glass Thermometer

Precautions

- Store a glass thermometer in a holder, because it is fragile and can break easily.
- Use cold water to clean a glass thermometer, because hot water will cause it to break.
- Use only a glass thermometer that is in perfect condition, not one that is chipped, cracked, or broken.

Preparation

1. Gather supplies
   - Thermometer
   - Thermometer holder
   - Cotton balls
   - Plastic trash bag
   - Paper towels
   - Soap
   ☐ ☐

Additional Information

1. You must wear disposable gloves to clean a rectal thermometer.

Fahrenheit thermometers are marked with alternating long and short lines. Every other long line is marked as an even degree, from 94 to 108 degrees. The other long lines are not marked. They are the odd degrees (95 to 107). The short lines between the long lines mark two tenths of a degree. An easy way to measure is to count by two's. For example, if the temperature reading is on the third short line past the long line that is marked 98, you would count "98 and two tenths, 98 and four tenths, 98 and six tenths." The temperature would be 98 and six tenths, or 98.6. The small arrow marks the average normal oral temperature.

2. Focus ☐ ☐

3. Knock and wait ☐ ☐

4. Introduce and identify ☐ ☐

5. Explain ☐ ☐

6. Place supplies ☐ ☐

7. Wash hands ☐ ☐

8. Gather and prepare ☐ ☐

9. Adjust bed ☐ ☐

10. Provide privacy ☐ ☐

Notes:

15

Completion

Additional Information

4. Clean the thermometer and put it away.

1. Ensure safety, comfort ☐ ☐

2. Put laundry in laundry bag ☐ ☐

3. Put disposables in trash bag ☐ ☐

4. Clean, put away equipment ☐ ☐

5. Say good-bye ☐ ☐

6. Dispose of trash bag ☐ ☐

7. Put laundry bag in hamper ☐ ☐

8. Wash hands ☐ ☐

9. Note, record, report ☐ ☐

_____

Student   Date

_____

Instructor   Date

Skill 6: Taking and Recording a Person's Oral Temperature with a Glass Thermometer

Precautions

- Never take an oral temperature if the person—
  Has had recent mouth surgery or has mouth disease.
  Is getting oxygen.
  Is short of breath or is having trouble breathing.
  Is confused or unconscious.
  Is paralyzed on one side of his body or face.
  Is breathing through his mouth instead of his nose.
  Has a tube in his nose.
  Is under 5 years of age.
- Use only a glass thermometer that is in perfect condition, not one that is chipped, cracked, or broken.

Preparation

1. Gather supplies
   - Clean oral thermometer (if the person does not have one at his bedside)
   - Thermometer sheath (optional)
   - Watch with a second hand
   - Disposable gloves (optional)
   - Cotton balls and tissues
   - Plastic trash bag
   - Paper towel
   - Pencil and paper to write down the temperature ☐ ☐

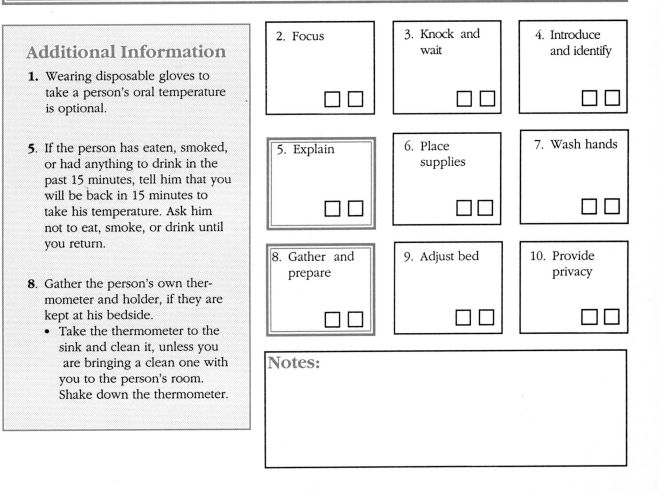

Additional Information

1. Wearing disposable gloves to take a person's oral temperature is optional.

5. If the person has eaten, smoked, or had anything to drink in the past 15 minutes, tell him that you will be back in 15 minutes to take his temperature. Ask him not to eat, smoke, or drink until you return.

8. Gather the person's own thermometer and holder, if they are kept at his bedside.
   - Take the thermometer to the sink and clean it, unless you are bringing a clean one with you to the person's room. Shake down the thermometer.

2. Focus ☐ ☐

3. Knock and wait ☐ ☐

4. Introduce and identify ☐ ☐

5. Explain ☐ ☐

6. Place supplies ☐ ☐

7. Wash hands ☐ ☐

8. Gather and prepare ☐ ☐

9. Adjust bed ☐ ☐

10. Provide privacy ☐ ☐

Notes:

Procedure

1. Put the thermometer sheath, if used, on the thermometer. ☐ ☐

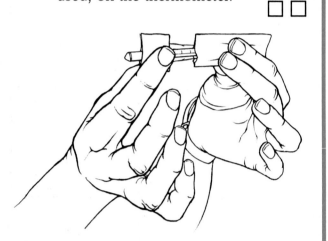

2. Put the bulb end of the thermometer under the person's tongue and slightly to one side. Ask the person to close her lips and not to bite down on the thermometer with her teeth. Help the person hold the thermometer in her mouth if necessary. Always stay with the person while you are taking an oral temperature. ☐ ☐

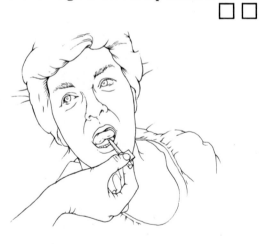

3. Note the time on your watch when you put the thermometer in the person's mouth, and keep the thermometer in place for 5 to 8 minutes. ☐ ☐

Why? With the oral method, 5 minutes is the *minimum* amount of time needed to measure the temperature accurately. ☐ ☐

4. Remove the thermometer from the person's mouth. Take off the thermometer sheath, if used, and throw it away in the plastic trash bag. If mucus or saliva on the thermometer makes it difficult to read, wipe off the thermometer with a tissue. ☐ ☐

5. Read the thermometer and place it on a clean, dry paper towel or tissue. ☐ ☐

Write down the temperature immediately on the paper that you brought with you. Be sure to write (O) for oral next to the number. Example: 98.6° F (O).

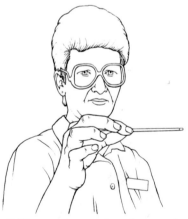

Why? You must write down the temperature immediately, because you may get distracted and forget the temperature before writing it on the official record.

Note: Remember to hold the thermometer at eye level while you read it.

Completion

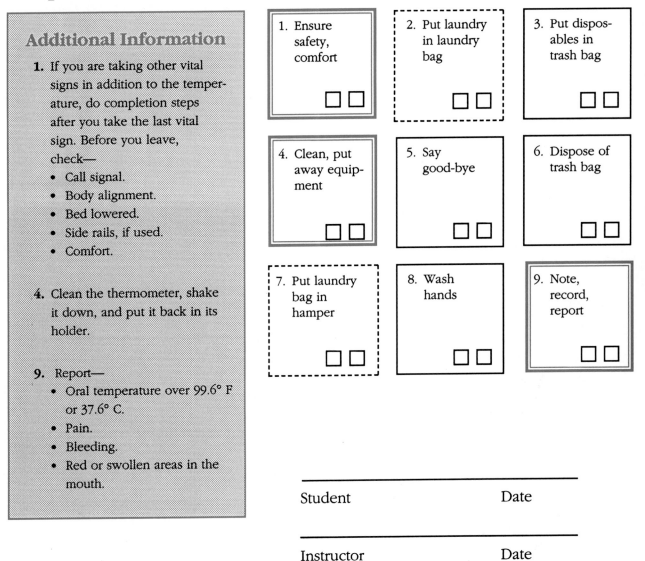

1. Ensure safety, comfort ☐ ☐

2. Put laundry in laundry bag ☐ ☐

3. Put disposables in trash bag ☐ ☐

4. Clean, put away equipment ☐ ☐

5. Say good-bye ☐ ☐

6. Dispose of trash bag ☐ ☐

7. Put laundry bag in hamper ☐ ☐

8. Wash hands ☐ ☐

9. Note, record, report ☐ ☐

_____   _____
Student   Date

_____   _____
Instructor   Date

Skill 7: Taking a Person's Rectal Temperature with a Glass Thermometer

Precautions

- Always use a rectal thermometer when taking a rectal temperature.
- Never take a rectal temperature if the person has—
  Diarrhea.
  A blocked rectum.
  Recently had a heart attack.
  Recently had rectal surgery or injury.
  Hemorrhoids.
- Use only a glass thermometer that is in perfect condition, not one that is chipped, cracked, or broken.

Preparation

1. Gather supplies
   - Rectal thermometer (if the person does not have one at his bedside)
   - Thermometer sheath (optional)
   - Lubricating jelly
   - Watch with a second hand
   - Plastic trash bag
   - Paper towels
   - Disposable gloves
   - Pencil and paper to write down the temperature ☐ ☐

Additional Information

5. Explain why you need to take a rectal temperature.

8. Gather the person's own rectal thermometer and holder, if they are kept at his bedside. Clean the thermometer. Shake down the thermometer.

9. The bed should be high enough so that you do not need to bend.

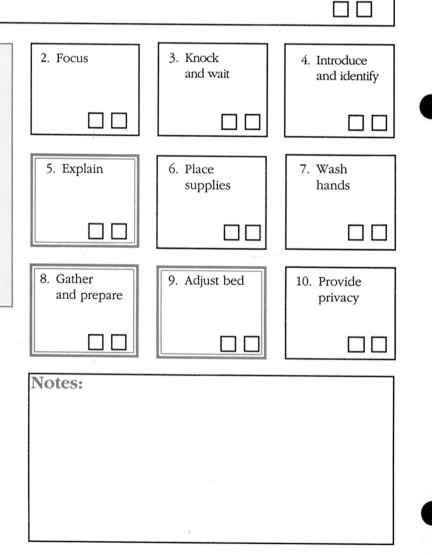

2. Focus ☐ ☐

3. Knock and wait ☐ ☐

4. Introduce and identify ☐ ☐

5. Explain ☐ ☐

6. Place supplies ☐ ☐

7. Wash hands ☐ ☐

8. Gather and prepare ☐ ☐

9. Adjust bed ☐ ☐

10. Provide privacy ☐ ☐

Notes:

Procedure

1. Put the thermometer sheath, if used, on the thermometer. Put the thermometer down on a clean paper towel or tissue. Have extra tissues within easy reach. ☐ ☐

2. Lower the side rail, if used, on the side where you will be working. ☐ ☐

3. Help the person lie on one side with his back toward you. Ask him to flex his top knee. Adjust his clothing and top covers so that he is covered. ☐ ☐

4. Put on disposable gloves. ☐ ☐

5. Put a small amount of lubricating jelly on a tissue. Use the lubricated tissue to make the bulb of the thermometer slippery, or insert the thermometer into a single-use envelope containing lubricant to lubricate the thermometer. ☐ ☐

Why? Lubricating the thermometer makes the procedure more comfortable for the person and reduces the chance of injury.

6. Turn back the top covers and adjust or remove clothing just enough so that you can see the anal area. ☐ ☐

Why? This helps to maintain privacy.

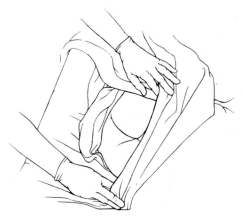

✓ 7. Lift the person's upper buttock and gently insert the bulb end of the thermometer into the anus, no more than 1 inch. ☐ ☐

Why? Inserting the thermometer more than 1 inch may injure rectal tissue.

8. Note the time on your watch when you put the thermometer in the person's rectum, and hold the thermometer in place for at least 3 minutes. ☐ ☐

Why? For the rectal method, 3 minutes is the *minimum* time required to obtain an accurate temperature reading.

Note: Always hold onto the thermometer while taking a rectal temperature.

9. Gently remove the thermometer and place it on a paper towel. Clean the anal area with a clean tissue. Take off the thermometer sheath, if it was used. Wipe off the thermometer with a tissue, if necessary. Throw the sheath and all tissues in the plastic trash bag. ☐ ☐

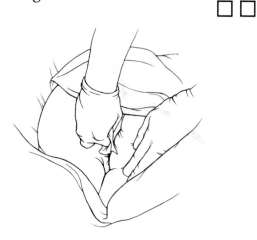

10. Read the thermometer and remember the number. ☐ ☐

11. Place the thermometer on a clean, dry paper towel or tissue. ☐ ☐

12. If gloves are soiled with feces, remove the gloves and throw them away in the plastic trash bag. ☐ ☐

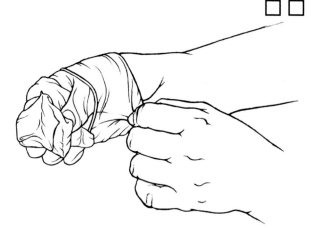

13. Write down the temperature immediately on the paper that you brought with you. Be sure to write (R) for rectal next to the temperature. Example: 99.6 ° F (R). ☐ ☐

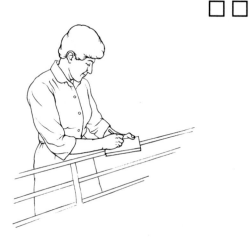

Completion

Additional Information

1. If you are taking other vital signs in addition to the person's temperature, do completion steps after you take the last vital sign. Before you leave, check—
- Call signal.
- Body alignment.
- Bed lowered.
- Side rails, if used.
- Comfort.

4. Clean the thermometer, shake it down, and put it back in its holder.

9. Report—
- Rectal temperature over 100.6° F or 38.1° C.
- Pain.
- Bleeding.
- Red or swollen areas.

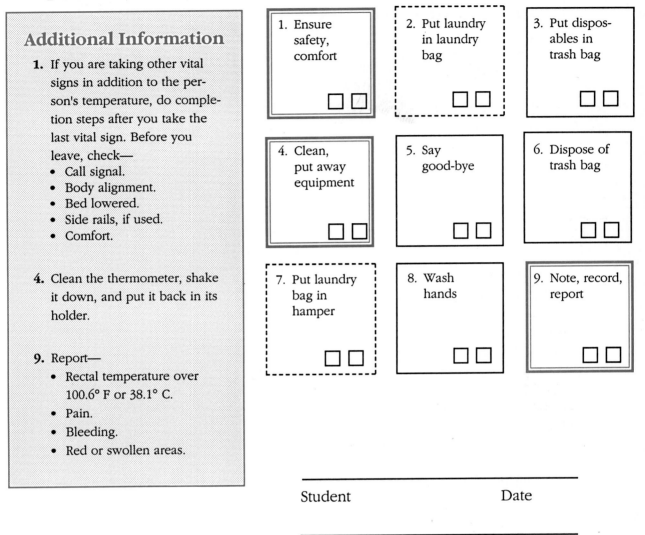

1. Ensure safety, comfort ☐ ☐

2. Put laundry in laundry bag ☐ ☐

3. Put disposables in trash bag ☐ ☐

4. Clean, put away equipment ☐ ☐

5. Say good-bye ☐ ☐

6. Dispose of trash bag ☐ ☐

7. Put laundry bag in hamper ☐ ☐

8. Wash hands ☐ ☐

9. Note, record, report ☐ ☐

_____
Student   Date

_____
Instructor   Date

Skill 8: Taking and Recording a Person's Axillary Temperature with a Glass Thermometer

Precautions

- Make sure the person is sitting or lying down during the procedure and not walking around with the thermometer under his arm.
- Use only a glass thermometer that is in perfect condition, not one that is chipped, cracked, or broken.

Preparation

1. Gather supplies
   - Clean thermometer (if the person does not have one at his bedside)
   - Thermometer sheath (optional)
   - Watch with a second hand
   - Cotton balls and tissues
   - Plastic trash bag
   - Paper towels
   - Pencil and paper to write down the temperature
   ☐ ☐

Additional Information

8. Gather the person's own thermometer and holder, if they are kept at his bedside.

Clean the thermometer and shake it down.

2. Focus
   ☐ ☐

3. Knock and wait
   ☐ ☐

4. Introduce and identify
   ☐ ☐

5. Explain
   ☐ ☐

6. Place supplies
   ☐ ☐

7. Wash hands
   ☐ ☐

8. Gather and prepare
   ☐ ☐

9. Adjust bed
   ☐ ☐

10. Provide privacy
   ☐ ☐

Notes:

Procedure

1. Put the thermometer sheath, if used, on the thermometer. ☐ ☐

2. Uncover the person's underarm area and dry it with a tissue, if necessary. Throw the tissue in the plastic trash bag. ☐ ☐

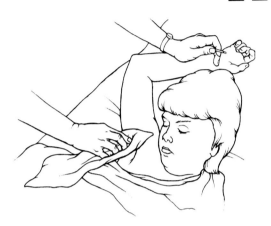

Why? Moisture from perspiration could change the temperature reading.

3. Put the bulb end of the thermometer in the middle of the person's underarm. ☐ ☐

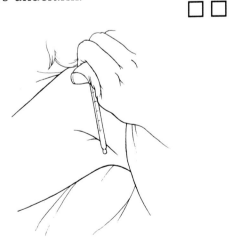

Bring her arm across his chest to hold the thermometer in place.

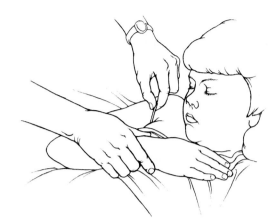

4. Note the time on your watch when you placed the thermometer under the person's arm, and keep the thermometer in place for at least 10 minutes. ☐ ☐

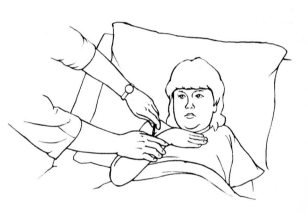

Why? For the axillary method, 10 minutes is the amount of time required for an accurate temperature reading.

Note: You will need to hold the thermometer in place for an infant or child, or if the person is unable to help. Always stay with the person while the thermometer is in place.

Skill 9: Using an Electronic Thermometer

Precautions
- Check to make sure equipment is working (electrically charged).

Preparation

1. Gather supplies
   - Electronic thermometer
   - Probe cover
   - Lubricating jelly (for rectal)
   - Disposable gloves (for rectal)
   - Plastic trash bag
   - Pencil and paper to write down the temperature ☐ ☐

Additional Information

1. Probes are detachable and will be coded to indicate whether they are rectal or oral/axillary.

9. Raise the bed when taking a rectal temperature.

2. Focus ☐ ☐

3. Knock and wait ☐ ☐

4. Introduce and identify ☐ ☐

5. Explain ☐ ☐

6. Place supplies ☐ ☐

7. Wash hands ☐ ☐

8. Gather and prepare ☐ ☐

9. Adjust bed ☐ ☐

10. Provide privacy ☐ ☐

Notes:

Procedure

1. Be sure that you have the appropriate probe. ☐ ☐

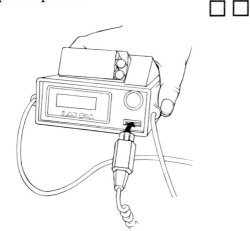

Turn the thermometer "on" by removing the probe from the location in the machine where it is stored (its "home" location). ☐ ☐

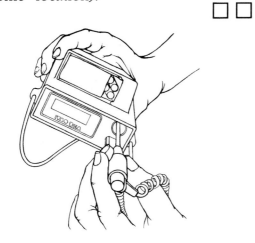

2. Insert the probe into the probe cover by pushing firmly until you feel the probe cover snap into place. ☐ ☐

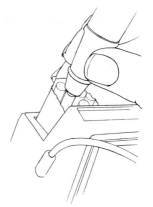

3. Position the person appropriately and place the covered probe into his mouth, under his arm, or into his rectum. Use disposable gloves when taking a rectal temperature, and before inserting it into the rectum. ☐ ☐

4. Read the number of the temperature on the small screen after the machine beeps. ☐ ☐

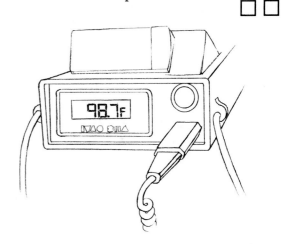

Note: The thermometer reading will flash while the temperature is registering. A beep will usually sound when the final temperature is registered.

Note: The final reading will hold steady for 5 minutes or until the probe is replaced into the machine.

5. Eject the probe cover and throw it into the plastic trash bag. Wipe the person's anal area with a tissue, if you took a rectal temperature, and throw away the tissue in the plastic trash bag. Take off the gloves, if you used them, and throw them into the plastic trash bag. Write down the temperature on the paper that you brought with you before returning the probe to its home. □ □

Completion

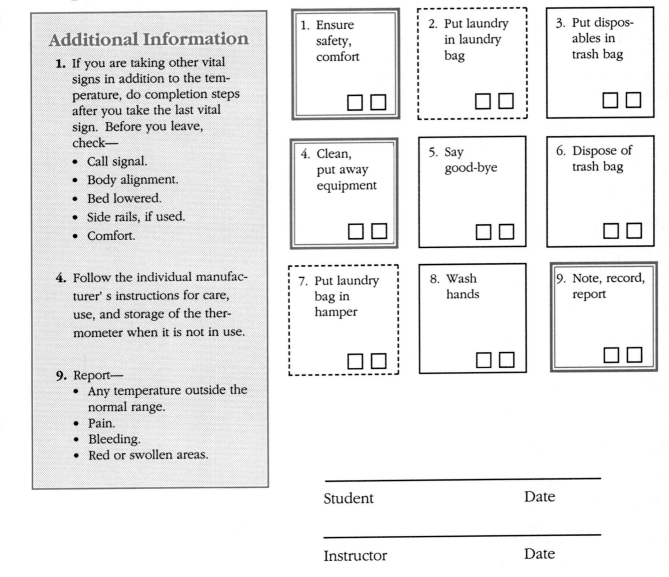

1. Ensure safety, comfort ☐ ☐	2. Put laundry in laundry bag ☐ ☐	3. Put disposables in trash bag ☐ ☐
4. Clean, put away equipment ☐ ☐	5. Say good-bye ☐ ☐	6. Dispose of trash bag ☐ ☐
7. Put laundry bag in hamper ☐ ☐	8. Wash hands ☐ ☐	9. Note, record, report ☐ ☐

_____

Student   Date

_____

Instructor   Date

Skill 10: Counting and Recording a Person's Pulse

Precautions

- Always use your fingers to take a person's radial pulse. Never take it with your thumb. The thumb has its own pulse, and you may count your pulse rate instead of the person's.
- Do not hold the person's arm up in the air when counting the radial pulse
- Be careful not to press too hard because this may make the radial pulse more difficult to feel.
- To take a person's apical pulse, place the person in a supine (on his back) or semi-Fowler's (sitting up with the head of the bed elevated for support) position.

Preparation

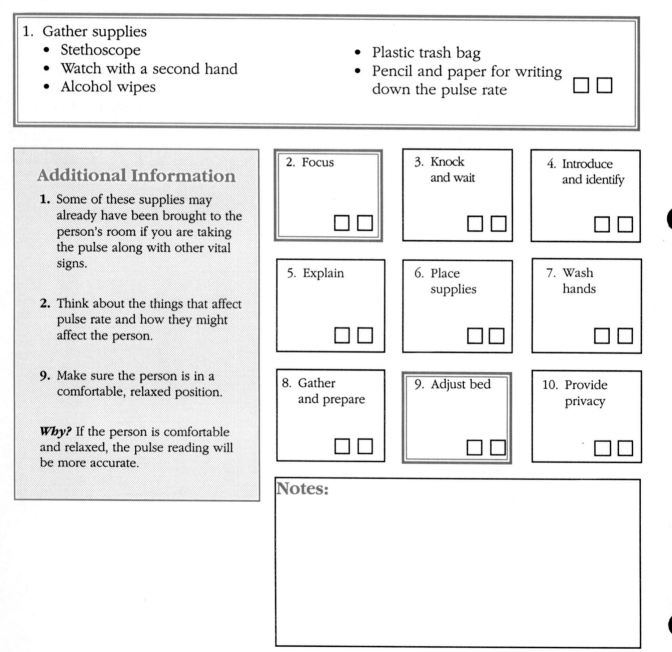

1. Gather supplies
   - Stethoscope
   - Watch with a second hand
   - Alcohol wipes
   - Plastic trash bag
   - Pencil and paper for writing down the pulse rate ☐ ☐

Additional Information

1. Some of these supplies may already have been brought to the person's room if you are taking the pulse along with other vital signs.

2. Think about the things that affect pulse rate and how they might affect the person.

9. Make sure the person is in a comfortable, relaxed position.

Why? If the person is comfortable and relaxed, the pulse reading will be more accurate.

2. Focus ☐ ☐

3. Knock and wait ☐ ☐

4. Introduce and identify ☐ ☐

5. Explain ☐ ☐

6. Place supplies ☐ ☐

7. Wash hands ☐ ☐

8. Gather and prepare ☐ ☐

9. Adjust bed ☐ ☐

10. Provide privacy ☐ ☐

Notes:

34

Procedure

Option 1: Radial Pulse

1. Gently press your first, second, and third fingers over the person's radial pulse. □ □

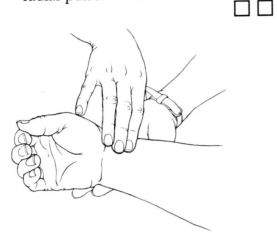

2. Using the second hand on your watch, count the number of beats for 1 minute. Until you are very comfortable with the skill, start counting when the second hand is at the "12" so that you do not lose track of when you started counting. □ □

3. While you count the pulse rate, note the rhythm and force, so that you can describe the pulse. □ □

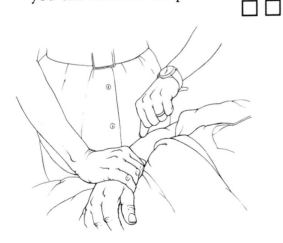

Why? A change in rhythm or force may indicate a problem. □ □

4. Write down the pulse rate on the paper that you brought with you. □ □

Why? You may become distracted and forget the rate before writing it on the official record.

Option 2: Apical Pulse

1. Place the person in a supine or semi-Fowler's position. □ □

2. Clean the earpieces and diaphragm of the stethoscope with an alcohol wipe and throw away the wipe in the plastic trash bag. □ □

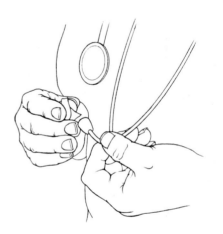

Why? Wiping off the ends of the stethoscope is an infection control measure.

3. Raise the person's gown or remove the clothing off his chest/nipple area on the left side. □ □

4. Warm the diaphragm of the stethoscope by warming it in your hand. □ □

5. Locate the apical pulse. The pulse point is located 2 to 3 inches to the left of the breastbone below the left nipple. ☐ ☐

6. Put the earpieces in your ears with the tips facing forward (toward your nose). ☐ ☐

7. Place the diaphragm over the pulse point. Hold it in place with your fingers, not your thumb, because you may hear the pulse in your thumb. ☐ ☐

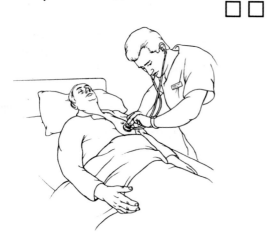

8. Count the pulse for 1 full minute. ☐ ☐ ●

9. Note any irregular beats, as well as the rhythm and the force, and write down the pulse rate and any irregularities on the paper that you brought with you. ☐ ☐

●

●

Completion

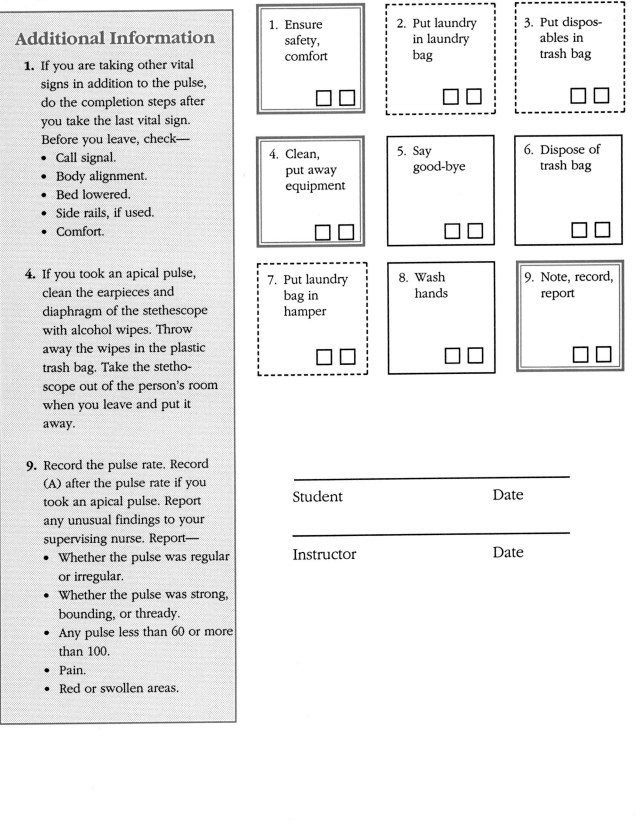

Student _____ Date

Instructor _____ Date

Skill 11: Counting and Recording a Person's Respirations

Precautions

- Always count respirations without the person being aware that you are counting them.

Preparation

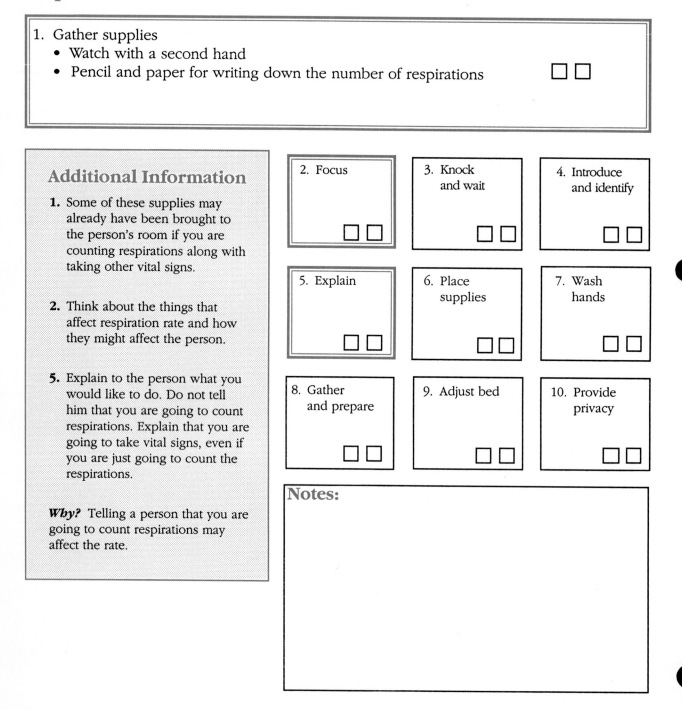

1. Gather supplies
   - Watch with a second hand
   - Pencil and paper for writing down the number of respirations   ☐ ☐

Additional Information

1. Some of these supplies may already have been brought to the person's room if you are counting respirations along with taking other vital signs.

2. Think about the things that affect respiration rate and how they might affect the person.

5. Explain to the person what you would like to do. Do not tell him that you are going to count respirations. Explain that you are going to take vital signs, even if you are just going to count the respirations.

Why? Telling a person that you are going to count respirations may affect the rate.

2. Focus   ☐ ☐

3. Knock and wait   ☐ ☐

4. Introduce and identify   ☐ ☐

5. Explain   ☐ ☐

6. Place supplies   ☐ ☐

7. Wash hands   ☐ ☐

8. Gather and prepare   ☐ ☐

9. Adjust bed   ☐ ☐

10. Provide privacy   ☐ ☐

Notes:

Procedure

1. Hold the person's wrist as if taking her radial pulse and count respirations by watching the rise and fall of her chest. One rise and one fall equals one respiration. Start when you see her chest rise. ☐ ☐

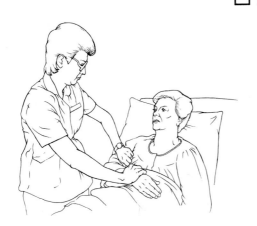

Why? When you appear to be taking her pulse, the person is less aware that you are observing the rise and fall of her chest.

2. Observe if the respirations are regular and if both sides of her chest rise equally. Also notice how deep they are and if the person seems to be having any pain or difficulty in breathing. ☐ ☐

3. Using the second hand on your watch, count respirations for 1 full minute. ☐ ☐

Note: If you wait until the second hand gets to the "12" each time you count, it makes it easier to keep track of how many seconds have gone by.

4. Write down the person's respiratory rate on the paper that you brought with you. ☐ ☐

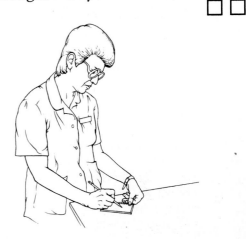

Why? You may get distracted and forget the rate before writing it on the official record.

Completion

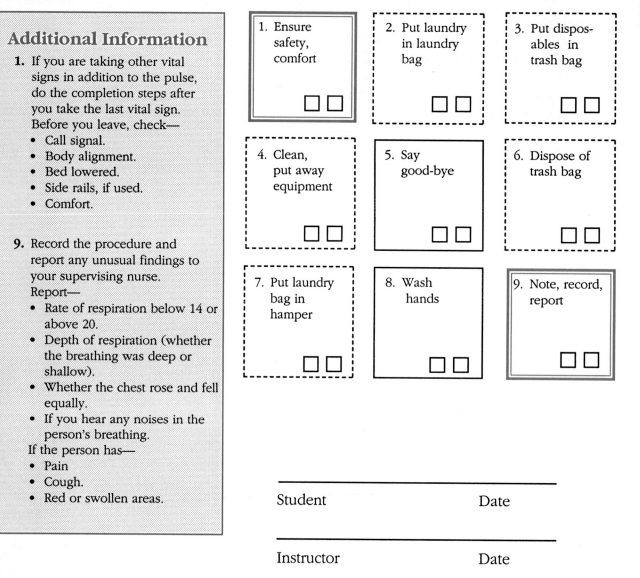

1. Ensure safety, comfort ☐ ☐

2. Put laundry in laundry bag ☐ ☐

3. Put disposables in trash bag ☐ ☐

4. Clean, put away equipment ☐ ☐

5. Say good-bye ☐ ☐

6. Dispose of trash bag ☐ ☐

7. Put laundry bag in hamper ☐ ☐

8. Wash hands ☐ ☐

9. Note, record, report ☐ ☐

_____
Student   Date

_____
Instructor   Date

Skill 12: Taking and Recording a Person's Blood Pressure

Precautions

- Put a cuff on a person's bare arm, and never put a cuff on a person's arm that has a cast or that has an IV (intravenous infusion) in place.
- Be careful about which arm you put the cuff on. For example, you should never put a cuff on an arm on the side where a woman has had a breast surgically removed (a mastectomy). You also should avoid putting a cuff on the weak arm of a person who has had a stroke. Ask your supervising nurse for instructions if the person has had both breasts removed or has paralysis in both arms.
- Always clean the earpieces and diaphragm of the stethoscope with alcohol before and after each use.
- Check the tubing and diaphragm of the stethoscope for cracks or holes.

Preparation

1. Gather supplies
   - Blood pressure machine (sphygmomano-meter) with the correct size cuff
   - Stethoscope
   - Alcohol wipes
   - Plastic trash bag
   - Pencil and paper to write down the BP reading ☐ ☐

Additional Information

1. Select the correct size cuff for the person, according to the following chart:

Arm Size	Cuff Size	Bladder Width
5-8 in	Child	3-4 in
7-10 in	Small adult	4 in
9-12 in	Adult	5-6 in
12-16 in	Large adult	6-7 in

2. Check the person's chart to find out what his blood pressure usually is. Also think about things that affect blood pressure and how these might affect the person.

8. Make sure that the person is seated or lying down, with his lower arm supported and his hand resting with the palm up. Assist the person in removing or adjusting clothing, as necessary, so that you can put the cuff on his bare skin.

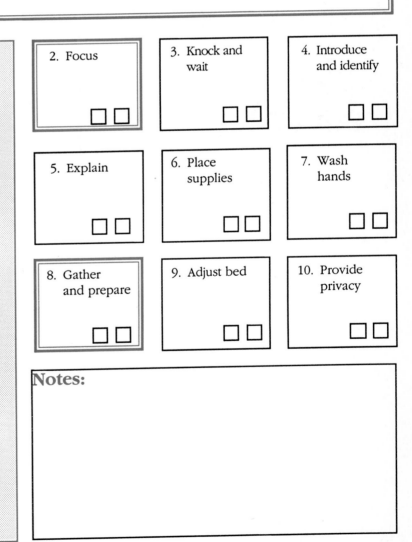

2. Focus ☐ ☐

3. Knock and wait ☐ ☐

4. Introduce and identify ☐ ☐

5. Explain ☐ ☐

6. Place supplies ☐ ☐

7. Wash hands ☐ ☐

8. Gather and prepare ☐ ☐

9. Adjust bed ☐ ☐

10. Provide privacy ☐ ☐

Notes:

Procedure

The three tasks for taking a person's blood pressure reading are as follows:

1. Positioning the blood pressure cuff
2. Palpating (feeling)
3. Auscultating (listening)

Task 1: Positioning the Blood Pressure Cuff

1. Locate the person's brachial pulse.

   □ □

2. Before putting the cuff on the person's arm, loosen the valve. If you turn the screw to the left, it opens the valve and lets the air escape from the bladder, which makes the cuff loose. If you turn the screw to the right, it closes the valve and keeps the air inside the bladder, which makes the cuff tight. A good way to remember this is by saying—

   □ □

"Left equals loose. Right equals tight."

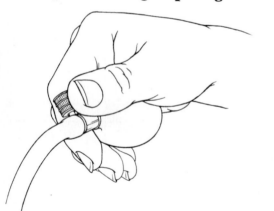

Turn the screw to the left and squeeze all the air out of the cuff.

3. Place the cuff on the person's upper arm, over bare skin, so that it is covering about two thirds of his upper arm. Put the center of the cuff's bladder 1 inch above his elbow on the inside of his arm over the brachial artery. To make sure the bladder is centered over the brachial artery, fold the bladder in half and place the fold over the artery. Or, if the cuff has an arrow, make sure the arrow is directly over the brachial artery.

   □ □

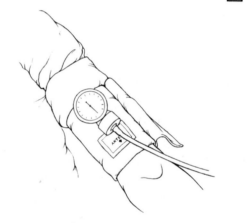

Why? Proper positioning is necessary to get an accurate reading.

4. Wrap the cuff around the person's arm snugly and smoothly so that the bladder presses evenly against his arm. Secure the cuff. Make sure it is snug enough to stay in place, but not uncomfortably tight.

   □ □

Why? The cuff must be wrapped smoothly to get an accurate reading.

Task 2: Palpating (feeling)

1. Feel the wrist (radial) pulse. ☐ ☐

2. Inflate the bladder by first tightening the valve (turn the screw to the right: right equals tight) and then pumping the bulb. Stop when you can no longer feel the pulse. Look at the gauge and note the reading. The number is an estimate of the systolic pressure. ☐ ☐

Note: Hold the bulb in one hand and use the fingers of that same hand to adjust the valve.

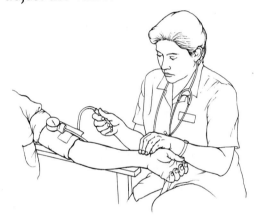

3. Let all the air out quickly. ☐ ☐

Why? Releasing the pressure of the cuff makes the person more comfortable.

4. Write down the reading immediately on the paper you brought with you. ☐ ☐

Why? You might get distracted and forget the number.

Task 3: Auscultating (listening)

1. Clean the earpieces and diaphragm of the stethoscope with an alcohol wipe, and throw away the wipe in the plastic trash bag. ☐ ☐

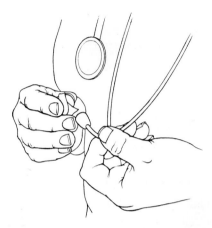

Why? Wiping off the ends of the stethoscope is an infection control measure.

2. Find the person's brachial pulse. ☐ ☐

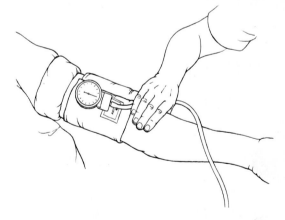

Why? The brachial pulse is the most convenient point in the body to measure blood pressure.

3. Put the earpieces in your ears with the tips facing forward (toward your nose). ☐ ☐

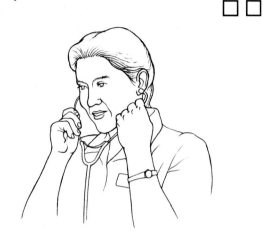

4. Place the diaphragm of the stethoscope firmly over the person's brachial pulse. Hold it in place with your fingers, not your thumb. You may feel the pulse in your thumb and be distracted from the visual reading. ☐ ☐

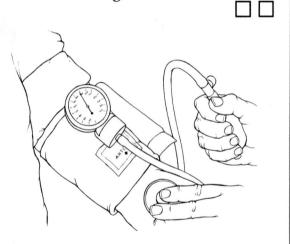

Note: Make sure the entire diaphragm is in contact with the person's skin.

5. Hold the rubber bulb in the other hand and, after tightening the valve (right equals tight), inflate the cuff quickly to 30 mm Hg above your estimated systolic pressure. ☐ ☐

6. Let the air out of the cuff slowly (left equals loose) at 2 to 4 mm each second. The reading when you first hear the pulse sound is the *systolic* pressure. Remember this number and continue letting the air out slowly. ☐ ☐

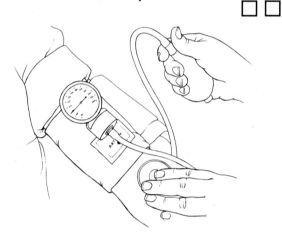

Why? Slowly releasing the air slows the speed at which the needle of the gauge or the mercury column falls, which makes it easier to note where the pulse sound starts and stops or changes.

7. The reading when the pulse sound stops or changes is the *diastolic* pressure. Remember this number and quickly let out the rest of the air. ☐ ☐

Note: If this reading is not noted the first time, wait at least 30 seconds to 1 minute and try again. Never try more than twice on one arm.

8. Immediately write down the systolic and diastolic readings on the paper that you brought with you. ☐ ☐

9. Remove the cuff from the person's arm. ☐ ☐

Completion

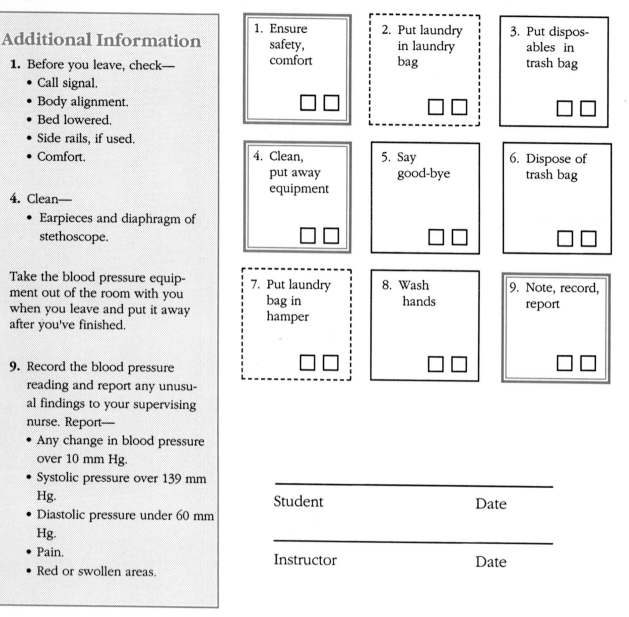

1. Ensure safety, comfort ☐ ☐

2. Put laundry in laundry bag ☐ ☐

3. Put disposables in trash bag ☐ ☐

4. Clean, put away equipment ☐ ☐

5. Say good-bye ☐ ☐

6. Dispose of trash bag ☐ ☐

7. Put laundry bag in hamper ☐ ☐

8. Wash hands ☐ ☐

9. Note, record, report ☐ ☐

_____
Student   Date

_____
Instructor   Date

Skill 13: Moving a Person Around in Bed

Precautions

- Assess the person and the room environment to determine your plan for moving him safely. Talk with your supervising nurse and check the care plan.
- Use proper body mechanics to prevent injury. To keep from injuring your back, always tighten your abdominal and buttocks muscles while positioning or transferring someone.
- Make sure bed brakes are locked.
- Ask a co-worker to help, if needed.

Preparation

1. Gather supplies
   Moving a person around in bed is most frequently done during the performance of another procedure. Think about the supplies you will need for that procedure and bring those. Be sure to bring the bed protectors. ☐ ☐

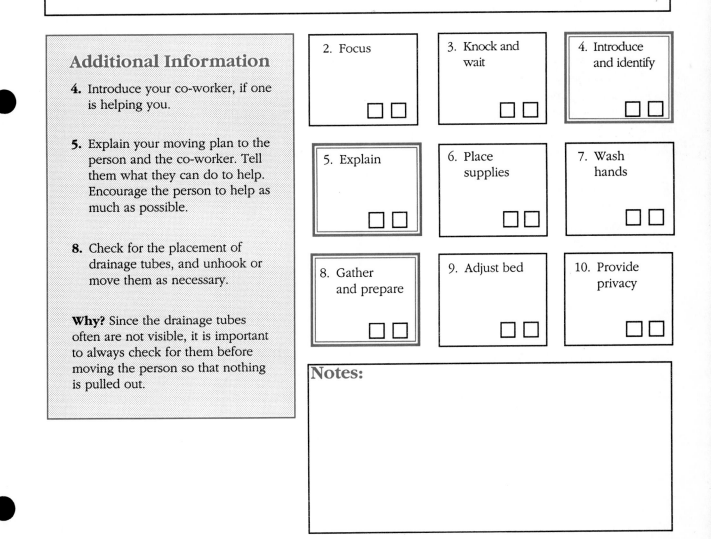

Additional Information

4. Introduce your co-worker, if one is helping you.

5. Explain your moving plan to the person and the co-worker. Tell them what they can do to help. Encourage the person to help as much as possible.

8. Check for the placement of drainage tubes, and unhook or move them as necessary.

Why? Since the drainage tubes often are not visible, it is important to always check for them before moving the person so that nothing is pulled out.

2. Focus ☐ ☐

3. Knock and wait ☐ ☐

4. Introduce and identify ☐ ☐

5. Explain ☐ ☐

6. Place supplies ☐ ☐

7. Wash hands ☐ ☐

8. Gather and prepare ☐ ☐

9. Adjust bed ☐ ☐

10. Provide privacy ☐ ☐

Notes:

Procedure

Option 1: Moving Up in Bed Using a Drawsheet (1 Nurse Assistant)

This procedure is used in home health situations where you may be alone and not have anyone to help you. To accomplish this procedure, you must be able to stand comfortably at the head of the bed. The bed must be pulled away from the wall and must *not* have a headboard. You cannot use proper body mechanics if you have to lean over a headboard.

1. Raise the height of the bed, if possible. ☐ ☐

Note: This decreases the amount you have to bend over.

2. Lower the side rail, if used, and loosen the drawsheet on one side of the bed. Raise the side rail and repeat this step on the other side of the bed. ☐ ☐

3. Make sure the person is lying as flat as possible. Ask the person to lift her head, or if she is unable, gently lift her head and remove the pillow. Place it alongside her or in a chair. ☐ ☐

Note: Lower the head of the bed as low as the person can tolerate.

4. Stand at the head of the bed with your feet 12 inches apart and one foot slightly behind the other. ☐ ☐

Note: Do not reach over a headboard.

5. Roll the top of the drawsheet close to the person's head and shoulders. Ask her to bend her knees if she is able and place her feet flat against the mattress so that she can help push up. ☐ ☐

6. With your palms up, grasp the rolled drawsheet with both hands, on either side of her head. ☐ ☐

Why? When you keep your palms up, you are able to lift better and avoid injury to your wrists.

7. Bend your hips and knees so that your upper back remains straight. ☐ ☐

8. Tell the person to get ready to move on the count of three. On the count of three, rock backward, pulling the drawsheet and the person up toward the head of the bed. ☐ ☐

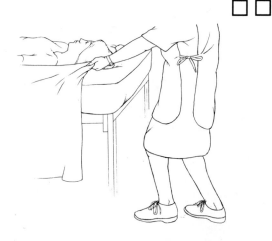

9. Help the person lift her head and replace the pillow for comfort. ☐ ☐

10. Retuck the drawsheet. ☐ ☐

11. Raise the side rail, if used. ☐ ☐

12. Lower the height of the bed. ☐ ☐

Option 2: Moving Up in Bed When the Person Can Help (One Nurse Assistant)

1. Raise the height of the bed, if possible. ☐ ☐

2. Lower the side rail, if used. ☐ ☐

3. Make sure the person is lying as flat as possible. Ask the person to lift her head or if she is unable, gently lift her head and remove the pillow. Place the pillow against the headboard. ☐ ☐

4. Stand with your feet about 12 inches apart. Point the toe of the foot nearest the headboard toward the headboard. ☐ ☐

5. Ask the person to bend her knees and place her feet firmly on the bed. Then ask her to place her hands palm side down on the bed. Place one arm under her shoulders and one hand under her buttocks. Ask her to help by pushing up with hands and feet on the count of three. ☐ ☐

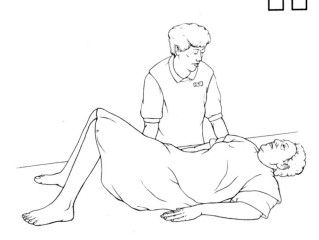

Or, if the person is able, ask him to reach back and hold onto the headboard with both hands. Ask him to assist you by pulling himself up on the count of three. ☐ ☐

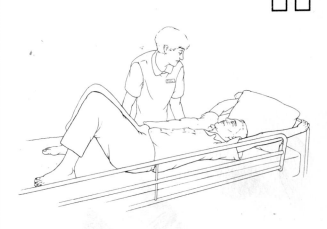

6. Count to three and, by shifting your weight onto the foot nearest the headboard, move the person toward the head of the bed. ☐ ☐

7. Repeat as necessary until the person is appropriately positioned. ☐ ☐

Note: Move the person only in short distances at one time so that you do not twist your back.

8. Gently lift the person's head and replace the pillow for comfort. ☐ ☐

9. Raise the side rail, if used. ☐ ☐

10. Lower the height of the bed. ☐ ☐

Option 3: Moving Up in Bed
(Two Nurse Assistants)

1. Tell your co-worker to stand on one side of the bed while you stand on the other side. Explain to your co-worker what to do. ☐ ☐

2. Lower both side rails, if used. ☐ ☐

3. Help the person lift her head and remove the pillow. Place it against the headboard. ☐ ☐

4. Make sure the person is lying as flat as possible in the *center* of the bed. ☐ ☐

5. Loosen the drawsheet on each side of the bed and roll it toward the side of the person until your hands are close to her body. Place a bed protector on the bed along each side of the person. ☐ ☐

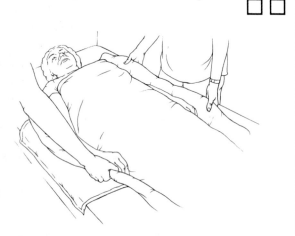

Why? By placing a bed protector on the bed, you avoid contaminating your uniform.

6. You and your co-worker stand as close to the bed as possible. Each of you lifts your knee that is facing the direction of the move (the one closest to the head-board) and places it on the bed on top of the bed protector. ☐ ☐

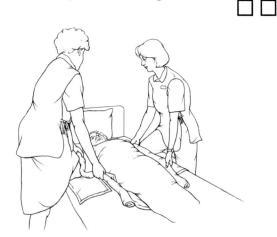

Note: Be sure the bed is in a lower-than-working-height position so that you can keep one foot firmly on the floor while your knee is on the bed.

7. Grasp the rolled-up drawsheet with your palms facing up. ☐ ☐

8. Tell the person that, if she is able to help, she should bend her knees and push up with her feet at the count of three. Tell your co-worker that on the count of three both of you together will move the person to the top of the bed by moving the drawsheet toward the headboard. ☐ ☐

9. On the count of three, gently lift the person to the top of the bed using the drawsheet to support most of his body. Lift her smoothly, without jerking, and lift her high enough off the bed so that she does not slide along the bottom sheet.

Why? If the person's skin rubs on the sheet, the friction can injure her skin.

Keep your elbows as close in to your body as you can to avoid straining your back. Shift your weight onto the knee that is on the bed as you lift. Repeat step nine until the person is correctly positioned at the top of the bed. ☐ ☐

Note: Move the person a little at a time rather than all the way up in one attempt so that you do not twist your back.

10. Gently lift the person's head and replace the pillow for comfort. ☐ ☐

11. Retuck the drawsheet. ☐ ☐

12. Raise the side rails, if used. ☐ ☐

Option 4: Moving to the Side of the Bed (One Nurse Assistant)

Note: Do not use this procedure if the person has a spinal cord injury or has had spinal surgery or spinal anesthesia.

1. Make sure the person is lying as flat as possible. ☐ ☐

2. If side rails are used, lower the one closer to you. ☐ ☐

3. Ask the person to lift her head, or if she is unable, gently lift her head and take away the pillow. Place it against the headboard. ☐ ☐

4. Stand with your feet 12 inches apart and one foot slightly behind the other. Bend your knees and keep your upper back as straight as possible. ☐ ☐

5. Ask the person to cross her arms over her chest. ☐ ☐

6. Place one arm under her neck and shoulders, and the other arm under her upper back. ☐ ☐

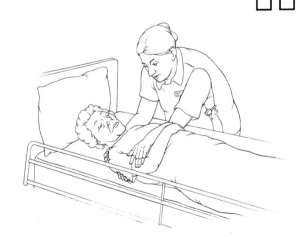

7. On the count of three, rock backwards and pull her upper body toward you. ☐ ☐

8. Reposition your hands, placing one hand under the person's waist and the other under her thighs. Using the same motion, count to three and rock backwards, pulling her lower body toward you. ☐ ☐

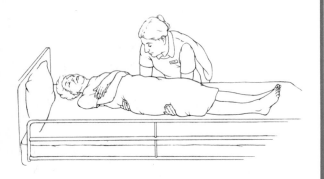

9. Finally, reposition your hands under her lower legs and feet and, on the count of three, move her legs and feet toward you. ☐ ☐

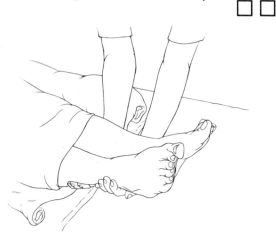

10. Help the person lift her head and replace the pillow for comfort. ☐ ☐

11. Raise the side rail, if used. ☐ ☐

Option 5: Moving to the Side of the Bed (Two Nurse Assistants)

1. Make sure the person is lying as flat as possible. ☐ ☐

2. Tell your co-worker to stand on one side of the bed while you stand on the other side. ☐ ☐

3. Lower both side rails, if used. ☐ ☐

4. Ask the person to lift her head, or if she is unable, gently lift the person's head and take away the pillow. Place it against the headboard. ☐ ☐

5. You will move the person away from yourself and toward your co-worker. Loosen the drawsheet on each side of the bed and roll it toward the side of person until your hands are close to her body. Put a bed protector on the bed alongside the person in front of you. ☐ ☐

6. Have your co-worker position his or her feet about 12 inches apart, with one foot slightly behind the other and the knees slightly bent.

Stand as close to the bed as possible, lift one knee, and place it on the bed on top of the bed protector, while keeping the other foot firmly on the floor. ☐ ☐

Note: Be sure the bed is in a lower-than-working-height position so that you can keep one foot firmly on the floor while your other knee is on the bed.

7. Both you and your co-worker grasp the rolled-up drawsheet with palms facing up. ☐ ☐

8. Tell your co-worker that on the count of three both of you together will move the person toward your co-worker's side of the bed by lifting the drawsheet. ☐ ☐

9. Tighten your abdominal and buttocks muscles and straighten your back. On the count of three, gently lift the person and move her to the side of the bed, using the drawsheet to support most of her body. Lift her smoothly, without jerking, and lift her high enough off the bed so that she does not slide along the bottom sheet. ☐ ☐

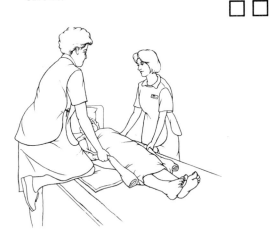

Note: You shift your weight from the foot on the floor to the knee on the bed as you lift.

Note: Your co-worker shifts his or her weight from the forward foot to the back foot as he or she lifts.

10. Help the person lift her head and replace the pillow for comfort. ☐ ☐

11. Retuck the drawsheet. ☐ ☐

12. Raise the side rails, if used. ☐ ☐

Option 6: Turning a Person (One or Two Nurse Assistants)

1. Tell your co-worker to stand on one side of the bed while you stand on the other side. ☐ ☐

2. Lower both side rails (or one side rail if you are turning the person by yourself). ☐ ☐

3. Ask the person to lift her head, or if she is unable, gently lift the person's head and remove the pillow. Place it against the headboard. ☐ ☐

4. Make sure the person is lying as flat as possible on one side of the bed, not in the center of the bed. If she is lying in the center of the bed, move her to the side following the steps in Option 4 or 5. ☐ ☐

5. Tell the person that she can help you by crossing her arms over her chest and crossing her ankles toward the direction that you are turning her. For example, if the person is turning onto her right side, have her put her left ankle on top of her right ankle. Assist her if necessary. ☐ ☐

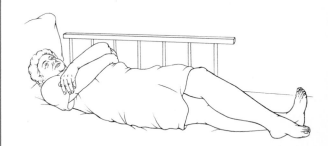

6. Stand on the side toward which the person is turning. Put a bed protector on the bed alongside the person. Stand as close to the bed as possible, lift one knee, and place it on the bed on top of the bed protector, while keeping the other foot firmly on the floor. Place one hand on the person's far shoulder and the other hand on her upper thigh. For example, if the person is turning onto her right side toward you, put your left hand on the person's left shoulder and your right hand on the person's left thigh. ☐ ☐

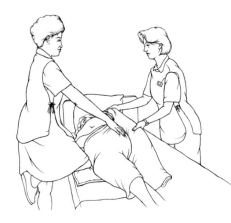

8. Help the person lift her head and replace the pillow for comfort. ☐ ☐

9. Raise the side rails, if used. ☐ ☐

Note: If you were turning the person by yourself, without the assistance of your co-worker, you would follow steps 2 through 5, and then roll her on her side toward you.

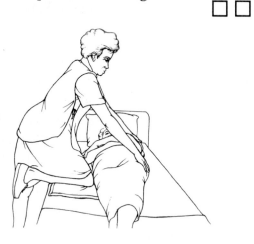

7. Your co-worker loosens the drawsheet and rolls it close to the side of the person's body. Grabbing the rolled-up drawsheet with palms up and using a broad base of support, your co-worker counts to three, lifts the drawsheet, and rolls the person onto her side. You help to roll her toward you by transferring your weight to your foot on the floor. ☐ ☐

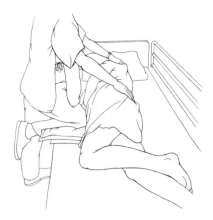

Note: Stand as close to the bed as possible. Be sure the bed is in a lower-than-working-height position so that you can keep one foot firmly on the floor.

Option 7: Lifting a Person's Head and Shoulders Off the Bed (One Nurse Assistant)

You may have to adjust a pillow or help someone sit up to readjust her clothing. To do this, you must raise the head and shoulders of the person off the bed.

1. Lower the side rail, if used. ☐ ☐

2. Stand on one side of the bed facing the head of the bed. Position your feet about 12 inches apart. ☐ ☐

3. If the person can help, ask her to place her arm that is nearer to you under your arm and to hold on behind your shoulder. ☐ ☐

4. Place your arm that is nearer to the person under her arm and behind her shoulder and your arm that is farther from the person under her upper back and shoulders. ☐ ☐

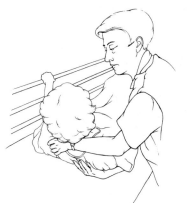

5. Raise the person's head and shoulders off the bed by shifting your weight toward the foot of the bed. Remember not to twist when you lift. Ask the person to assist you as much as she can by helping to support herself with her free hand. Use your hand that is under her shoulders to readjust the pillow. ☐ ☐

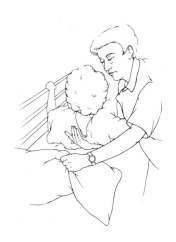

Completion

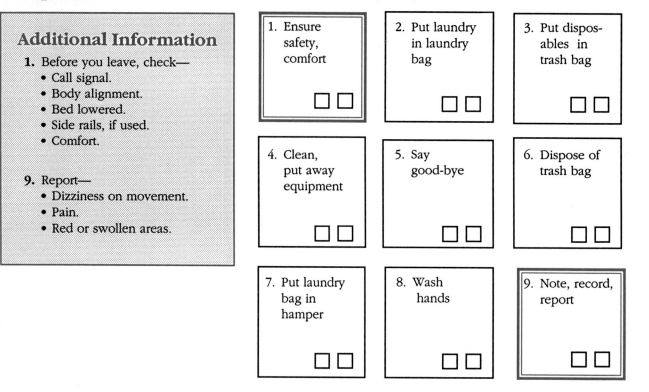

1. Ensure safety, comfort ☐ ☐	2. Put laundry in laundry bag ☐ ☐	3. Put disposables in trash bag ☐ ☐
4. Clean, put away equipment ☐ ☐	5. Say good-bye ☐ ☐	6. Dispose of trash bag ☐ ☐
7. Put laundry bag in hamper ☐ ☐	8. Wash hands ☐ ☐	9. Note, record, report ☐ ☐

_____

Student   Date

_____

Instructor   Date

Skill 14: Positioning a Person in a Supine Position

Precautions

- Assess the person and the room environment to determine your plan for moving him safely. Talk with your supervising nurse and check the care plan.
- Use proper body mechanics. To avoid injuring your back, always tighten your abdominal and buttocks muscles while positioning or transferring someone.
- Make sure bed brakes are locked.
- Ask a co-worker to help, if needed.

Preparation

1. Gather supplies
   - Pillows
   - Rolled blanket or towels
   - Foot support ☐ ☐

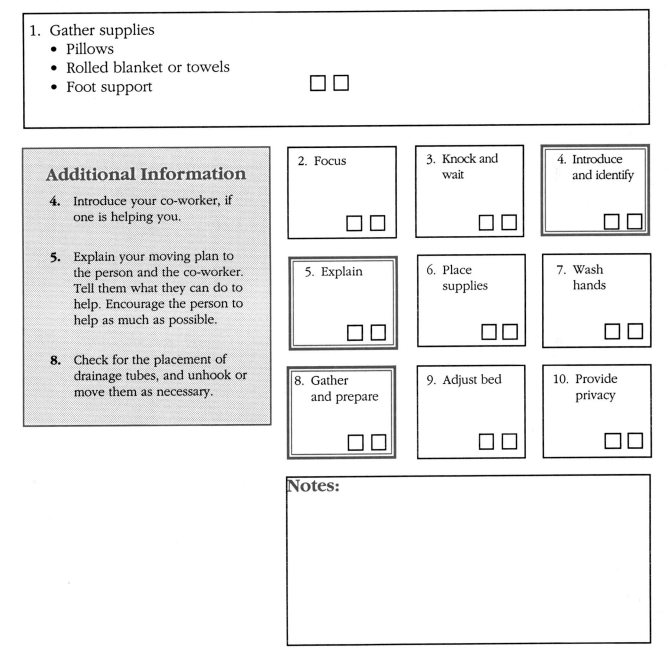

Additional Information

4. Introduce your co-worker, if one is helping you.

5. Explain your moving plan to the person and the co-worker. Tell them what they can do to help. Encourage the person to help as much as possible.

8. Check for the placement of drainage tubes, and unhook or move them as necessary.

2. Focus ☐ ☐

3. Knock and wait ☐ ☐

4. Introduce and identify ☐ ☐

5. Explain ☐ ☐

6. Place supplies ☐ ☐

7. Wash hands ☐ ☐

8. Gather and prepare ☐ ☐

9. Adjust bed ☐ ☐

10. Provide privacy ☐ ☐

Notes:

Procedure

1. If necessary, lower the head and foot of the bed to make it flat. □ □

2. Lower the side rail, if used, on the side where you are working. □ □

3. If drainage tubes are used, unhook or move them, as necessary. □ □

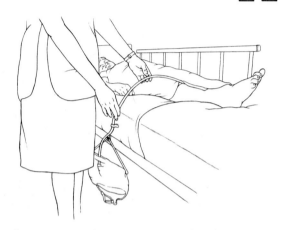

4. Position the person so that he is lying on his back in the center of the bed. □ □

5. Place him in proper body alignment. In the supine position, his body is in alignment when—

   • His head is supported with a pillow.
   • His arms are extended and, if there is paralysis or weakness, they are supported by small pillows so that his hand is higher than his elbow and shoulder. This position improves blood return to the heart. If a person is unable to move his hands, position his palms so that they face down.

   • His thighs are in a straight line from his hips.

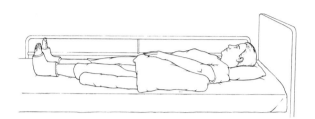

Note: Use a small cushion or rolled towel to support the small of his back.

Note: If the person's foot tends to roll outward, place a rolled towel or pillow against his outer thighs.

Note: Use a splint or foot board to keep his toes pointing upward. To keep pressure off his heels, use a small pad under his calves and ankles.

6. Raise the side rail, if used. □ □

Completion

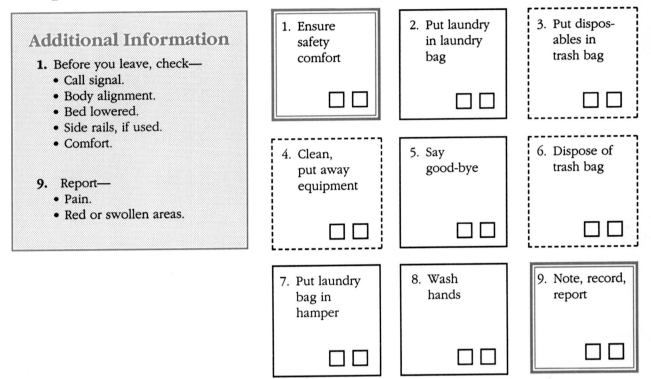

1. Ensure safety comfort ☐ ☐

2. Put laundry in laundry bag ☐ ☐

3. Put disposables in trash bag ☐ ☐

4. Clean, put away equipment ☐ ☐

5. Say good-bye ☐ ☐

6. Dispose of trash bag ☐ ☐

7. Put laundry bag in hamper ☐ ☐

8. Wash hands ☐ ☐

9. Note, record, report ☐ ☐

_____   _____
Student   Date

_____   _____
Instructor   Date

Skill 15: Positioning a Person in a Fowler's Position

Precautions

- Assess the person and the room environment to determine your plan for moving him safely. Talk with your supervising nurse and check the care plan.
- Use proper body mechanics. To keep from injuring your back, always tighten your abdominal and buttock muscles while positioning or transferring someone.
- Make sure bed brakes are locked.
- Ask a co-worker for help, if needed.

Preparation

1. Gather supplies
   Bring these supplies to the person's room
   - Pillows
   - Rolled blanket or towel
   - Foot support ☐ ☐

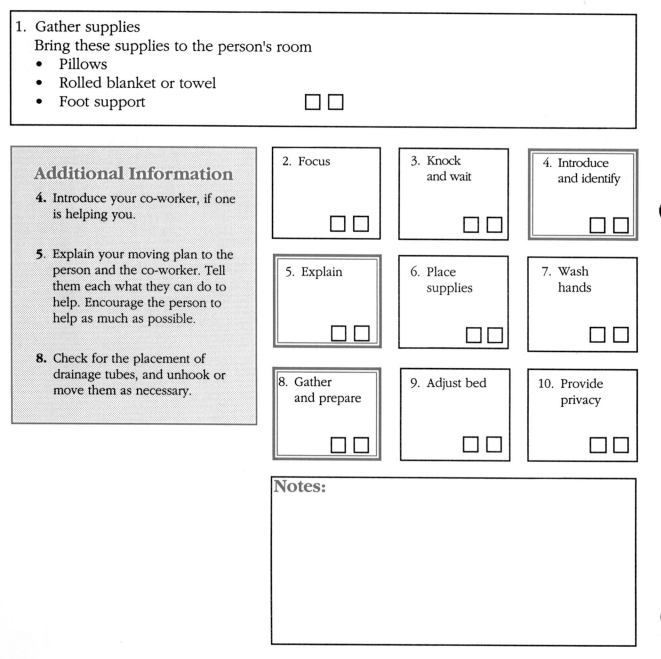

Additional Information

4. Introduce your co-worker, if one is helping you.

5. Explain your moving plan to the person and the co-worker. Tell them each what they can do to help. Encourage the person to help as much as possible.

8. Check for the placement of drainage tubes, and unhook or move them as necessary.

2. Focus ☐ ☐

3. Knock and wait ☐ ☐

4. Introduce and identify ☐ ☐

5. Explain ☐ ☐

6. Place supplies ☐ ☐

7. Wash hands ☐ ☐

8. Gather and prepare ☐ ☐

9. Adjust bed ☐ ☐

10. Provide privacy ☐ ☐

Notes:

Procedure

1. Lower the side rails, if used, on the side where you are working. ☐ ☐

2. Make sure the person is supine, in the center of the bed, and remove all pillows. Raise the head of the bed 90 degrees for high Fowler's position, 45 degrees for Fowler's position, and 30 degrees for semi-Fowler's or low Fowler's position. Replace the pillows. ☐ ☐

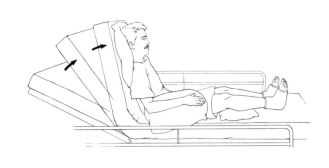

Note: A person sitting up in bed is in *Fowler's position.*

3. Raise the foot of the bed very slightly, just enough to prevent the person from sliding down in the bed. (Or, place a pillow or folded blanket under his legs.) Make sure the person is in proper body alignment. ☐ ☐

4. If the person has a weak forearm and wrist, support them with a pillow, keeping the wrist higher than the elbow. If the person is unable to move his hands, position them so that his palms face down. ☐ ☐

Why? The forearm and wrist must be elevated when the person's arm is weak or paralyzed to aid the return of blood to his heart and to prevent swelling of his hand.

5. Place a foot support, if needed. ☐ ☐

Why? Maintaining proper position of the person's feet prevents "foot drop." Foot drop causes the toes to drop downward. Then, the person is unable to bring his foot up into a normal walking position.

Note: Some people may have forearm, wrist, hand, or foot splints to keep their bodies in proper alignment. If a person uses splints, check to see that they are properly applied and that they are clean and dry.

6. Raise the side rail, if used. ☐ ☐

Completion

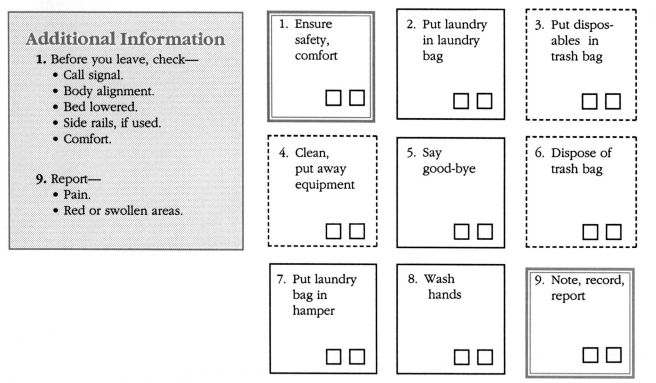

1. Ensure safety, comfort ☐ ☐

2. Put laundry in laundry bag ☐ ☐

3. Put disposables in trash bag ☐ ☐

4. Clean, put away equipment ☐ ☐

5. Say good-bye ☐ ☐

6. Dispose of trash bag ☐ ☐

7. Put laundry bag in hamper ☐ ☐

8. Wash hands ☐ ☐

9. Note, record, report ☐ ☐

_____

Student   Date

_____

Instructor   Date

Skill 16: Positioning a Person in a Modified Side-Lying (Lateral) Position

Precautions

- Assess the person and the room environment to determine your plan for moving him safely. Talk with your supervising nurse and check the care plan.
- Use proper body mechanics. To keep from injuring your back, always tighten your abdominal and buttock muscles while positioning or transferring someone.
- Make sure bed brakes are locked.
- Ask a co-worker for help, if needed.

Preparation

1. Gather supplies
   - Pillows
   - Rolled blanket or towel
   - Bed protector ☐ ☐

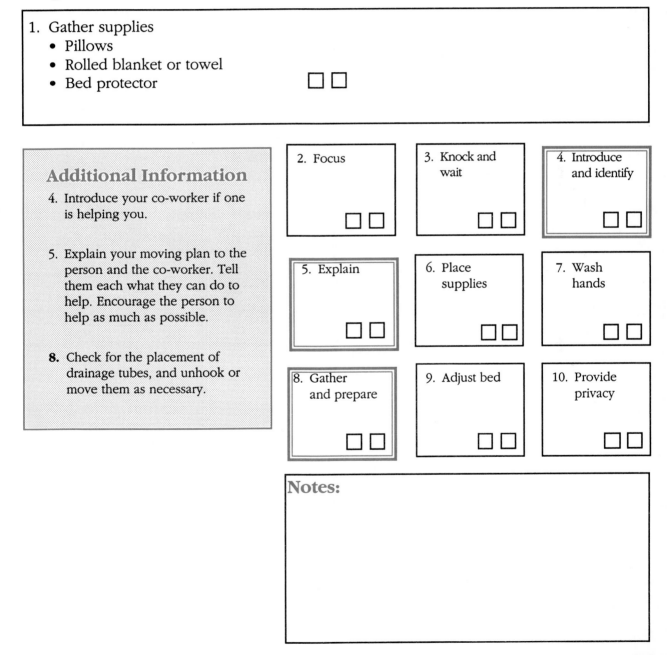

Additional Information

4. Introduce your co-worker if one is helping you.

5. Explain your moving plan to the person and the co-worker. Tell them each what they can do to help. Encourage the person to help as much as possible.

8. Check for the placement of drainage tubes, and unhook or move them as necessary.

2. Focus ☐ ☐

3. Knock and wait ☐ ☐

4. Introduce and identify ☐ ☐

5. Explain ☐ ☐

6. Place supplies ☐ ☐

7. Wash hands ☐ ☐

8. Gather and prepare ☐ ☐

9. Adjust bed ☐ ☐

10. Provide privacy ☐ ☐

Notes:

Procedure

1. Lower the side rail, if used, on the side where you are working. ☐ ☐

2. Make sure the bed is as flat as possible. ☐ ☐

3. Ask the person to help with the move by crossing her arms and ankles toward the direction you are turning her. ☐ ☐

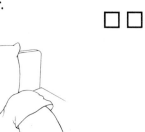

4. Following the procedure for moving a person to the side of the bed, and with the assistance of your co-worker, move the person to the far side of the bed, away from the direction she will be facing. ☐ ☐

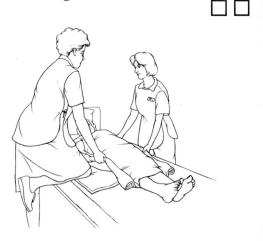

5. Turn the person onto her side so that she is off her coccyx (tail bone), but not directly on her hip, by doing the following: ☐ ☐

If you are on the side toward which the person is turning, place a bed protector on the bed and put one knee on it. Keep your other foot firmly on the floor. Place one hand on her shoulder and the other hand on her upper thigh. For example, if the person is turning onto her right side toward you, put your left hand on her left shoulder and your right hand on her left thigh.

6. Your co-worker loosens the draw-sheet and rolls it up close to the person's body. She grabs the drawsheet with the palms up. Using a broad base of support, she counts to three, lifts the draw-sheet, and rolls the person onto her side, while you help to roll her toward you. ☐ ☐

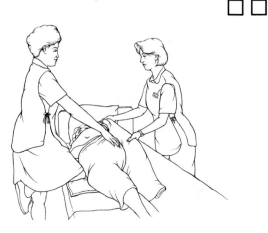

Note: Your co-worker keeps her body close to the bed and her knees slightly flexed.

7. Position the person in proper body alignment:

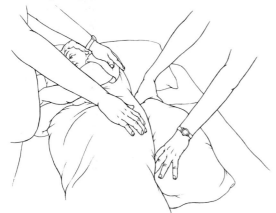

- Support her head with a pillow.
- Adjust her shoulder so that she is not lying on her arm.
- Support her back with a rolled blanket or towel to keep her in proper position.
- Support her top arm with a pillow.
- Flex her top knee.

- Place her top leg forward and support it with pillows so that it does not rest on top of her lower leg and does not pull on the hip joint.
- If the person is wearing alignment splints, check to make sure they are properly applied and that they are clean and dry. ☐ ☐

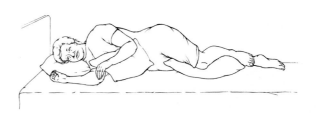

8. Retuck the drawsheet. ☐ ☐

9. Raise the side rail, if used. ☐ ☐

Completion

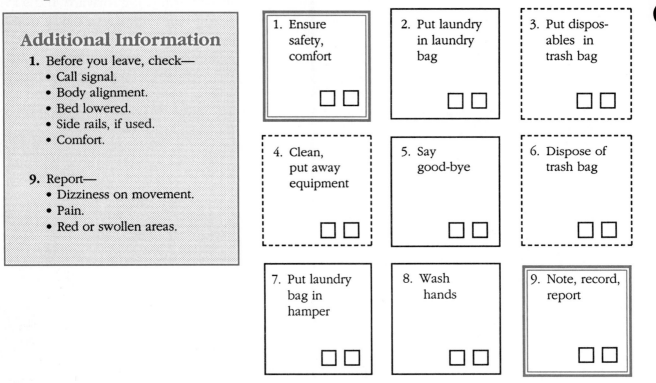

1. Ensure safety, comfort ☐ ☐

2. Put laundry in laundry bag ☐ ☐

3. Put disposables in trash bag ☐ ☐

4. Clean, put away equipment ☐ ☐

5. Say good-bye ☐ ☐

6. Dispose of trash bag ☐ ☐

7. Put laundry bag in hamper ☐ ☐

8. Wash hands ☐ ☐

9. Note, record, report ☐ ☐

_____

Student   Date

_____

Instructor   Date

Skill 17: Positioning a Person in a Prone Position

Precautions

When you help someone lie on his stomach, you help him into the prone position. This position is not often used, because many people find it uncomfortable and it often requires a physician's order.

- Assess the person and the room environment to determine your plan for moving him safely. Talk with your supervising nurse and check the care plan.
- Use proper body mechanics. To avoid injuring your back, always tighten your abdominal and buttocks muscles while positioning or transferring someone.
- Make sure the bed brakes are locked.
- Ask a co-worker to help, if needed.

Preparation

1. Gather supplies
   - Bed protector
   - Rolled blanket or towel
   ☐ ☐

Additional Information

4. Introduce your co-worker, if one is helping you.

5. Explain your moving plan to the person and the co-worker. Tell them what they can do to help. Encourage the person to help as much as possible.

8. Check for the placement of drainage tubes, and unhook or move them as necessary.

2. Focus ☐ ☐	3. Knock and wait ☐ ☐	4. Introduce and identify ☐ ☐
5. Explain ☐ ☐	6. Place supplies ☐ ☐	7. Wash hands ☐ ☐
8. Gather and prepare ☐ ☐	9. Adjust bed ☐ ☐	10. Provide privacy ☐ ☐

Notes:

Procedure

1. Lower the side rail, if used, on the side of the bed where you are working. ☐ ☐

2. Make sure the person is lying as flat as possible. ☐ ☐

3. Gently lift the person's head and remove her pillow. ☐ ☐

4. Tell the person that she can help to roll over, if she is able. ☐ ☐

5. With the help of your co-worker, follow the procedure for moving a person to the side of the bed. ☐ ☐

6. Put one hand on her far shoulder and one hand on her far hip and your knee on top of a bed protector on the bed. ☐ ☐

Note: Be sure the arm close to you is tucked close to the person or extended up along side her head so that it will not be trapped or caught under her body when she rolls over. Tuck a folded blanket or small pillow alongside her upper abdomen.

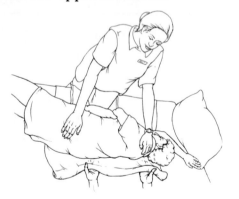

7. Your co-worker loosens the drawsheet, grabs it with her palms up, and rolls it close to the person's body. Using a broad base of support, she counts to three, lifts the drawsheet, and rolls the person, while you gently turn her toward you and onto her stomach with her head turned to the side. ☐ ☐

8. Position the person in proper body alignment:
   - Help her move down slightly so that her feet are over the end of the mattress or place a pillow under her shins to raise his toes off the bed.

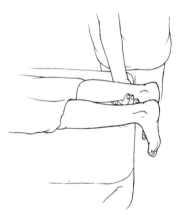

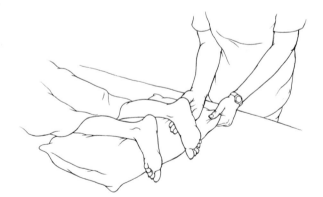

Use the drawsheet, if necessary, to move her down in the bed.

- Place a small pillow or folded blanket under her head, and adjust the one under her upper abdomen.
- Place the arm the person is facing with the elbow bent at a 90-degree angle at her side and her other arm straight along the other side. □ □

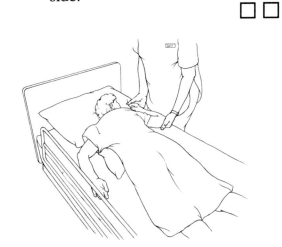

9. Retuck the drawsheet. □ □

10. Raise the side rail, if used. □ □

Completion

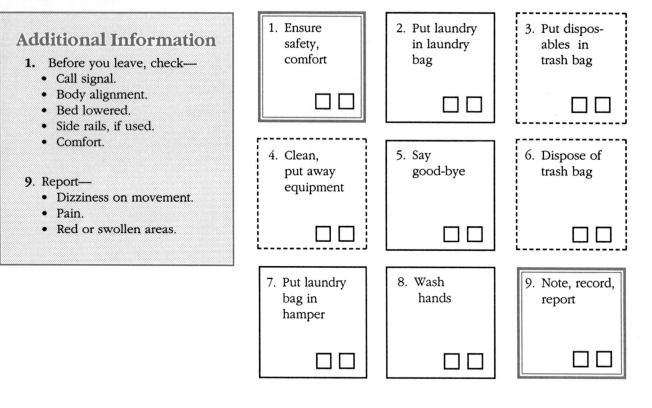

1. Ensure safety, comfort ☐ ☐

2. Put laundry in laundry bag ☐ ☐

3. Put disposables in trash bag ☐ ☐

4. Clean, put away equipment ☐ ☐

5. Say good-bye ☐ ☐

6. Dispose of trash bag ☐ ☐

7. Put laundry bag in hamper ☐ ☐

8. Wash hands ☐ ☐

9. Note, record, report ☐ ☐

_____

Student   Date

_____

Instructor   Date

Skill 18: Transferring a Person from the Bed to a Chair

Precautions

- Assess the person and room environment to determine your plan for transferring him safely. Talk with your supervising nurse or check the care plan.
- Use proper body mechanics. To keep from injuring your back, always tighten your abdominal and buttock muscles while positioning or transferring someone.
- Make sure bed brakes are locked.
- Ask a co-worker to help, if needed.
- Do not use a safety belt if the person has:
  - Had recent abdominal, chest, or back surgery.
  - Severe respiratory problems.
  - Severe cardiac problems.

Preparation

1. Gather supplies
   - Safety belt (transfer belt or walking belt with handles) if you are using one ☐ ☐

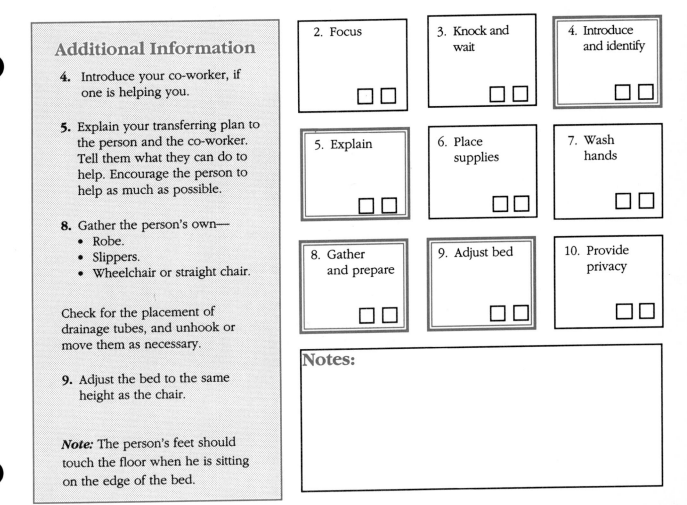

Additional Information

4. Introduce your co-worker, if one is helping you.

5. Explain your transferring plan to the person and the co-worker. Tell them what they can do to help. Encourage the person to help as much as possible.

8. Gather the person's own—
   - Robe.
   - Slippers.
   - Wheelchair or straight chair.

   Check for the placement of drainage tubes, and unhook or move them as necessary.

9. Adjust the bed to the same height as the chair.

Note: The person's feet should touch the floor when he is sitting on the edge of the bed.

2. Focus ☐ ☐

3. Knock and wait ☐ ☐

4. Introduce and identify ☐ ☐

5. Explain ☐ ☐

6. Place supplies ☐ ☐

7. Wash hands ☐ ☐

8. Gather and prepare ☐ ☐

9. Adjust bed ☐ ☐

10. Provide privacy ☐ ☐

Notes:

Procedure

1. Place the wheelchair or stationary chair at a slight angle against the bed on the person's stronger side. ☐ ☐

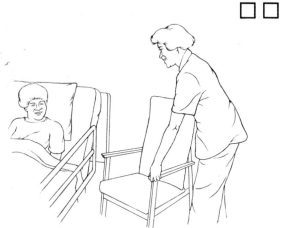

2. Lock the bed brakes. If a wheelchair is used, remove or fold back the wheelchair footrests, and lock the brakes. ☐ ☐

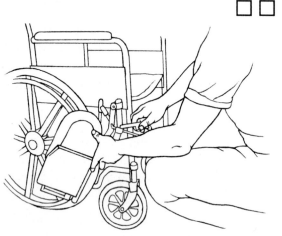

3. Raise the head of the bed so that the person is almost in a sitting position. ☐ ☐

4. Lower the side rail, if used, that is nearer to the wheelchair. ☐ ☐

5. With your knees bent and back straight, put one of your arms under the person's shoulders and the other arm under her thighs. Do not twist your back at the waist. If a co-worker is helping, one nurse assistant holds the person with one hand under the person's arm and around her shoulder and the other nurse assistant uses both hands to support her legs. ☐ ☐

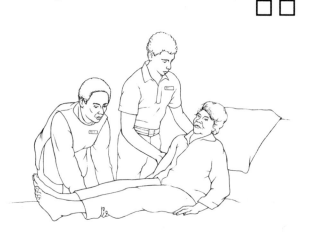

6. Turn the person toward you into a sitting position, bringing her legs to a dangling position over the side of the bed. ☐ ☐

Note: Stay with her and encourage her to sit on the side of the bed for 2 minutes before going on with the procedure. Some dizziness is common when a person sits up after being in bed for a while. See if it passes in 2 minutes. If it doesn't pass, if it gets worse, if she becomes sweaty or short of breath, or if she is in any pain, lay her back down, raise the side rail, if used. Report the situation to your supervising nurse.

7. Help the person put on her clothing, including footwear. ☐ ☐

Option 1: One Nurse Assistant, Without a Safety Belt, When the Person Can Help

To safely transfer a person by yourself without a safety belt, the person must need only steadying and minimal support. She must be able to stand with support, must be able to pivot, and must be predictable.

1. Tell the person you are going to put your arms under her arms and that she must put her arms around your waist or shoulders, not your neck. Placing arms around a caregiver's neck can injure the caregiver. Have the person raise her arms, then place your arms under her arms, holding on to her shoulders. Have her place her arms around your waist or shoulders as she leans forward. ☐ ☐

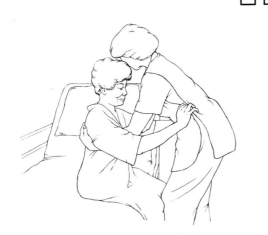

Note: When she gets ready to move, her buttocks should be at the edge of the bed so that she can keep her balance when you shift her weight forward. Her feet should be flat on the floor and her heels pointed slightly toward the direction of the move. This helps to keep her feet from becoming tangled when pivoting to the chair.

2. Place one foot facing the person with your knee (the one farther from the chair) between her knees and your other foot in the direction of the move. Bend your knees, tighten your abdominal and buttocks muscles, and keep your back straight. ☐ ☐

Note: Get as close as possible in a "hugging position." Remember to use proper body mechanics—use a good base of support, keep the person close, keep your back straight, lift smoothly, do not jerk, and do not twist. Put your head to the person's side closest to the chair so that you can keep it in sight during the move.

Note: Do not put pressure under the person's arms.

3. Tell the person that on the count of three you are going to assist her to a standing position. Rock back and forth gently on each count to create momentum and, on the count of three, raise her to a standing position. Turn your body with her as she pivots until she is right in front of the wheelchair. Ask her to tell you when she can feel the chair against the back of her legs. ☐ ☐

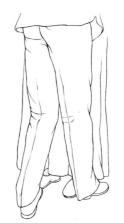

4. Lower her into the chair by bending your knees and keeping your back straight. ☐ ☐

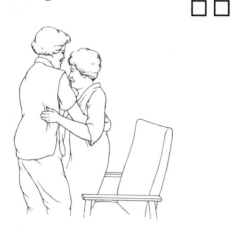

She can help by placing her hands on the chair arms and helping to lower herself into the chair.

Option 2: One Nurse Assistant, with a Safety Belt, When the Person Can Help

To safely transfer a person by yourself with a safety belt, the person must be able to stand with support, must be able to pivot, and must be predictable.

1. Stand in front of the person, facing her, and put the safety belt around her waist. The belt should be snug but not tight. She should be sitting with her buttocks on the edge of the bed, her feet flat on the floor, and her heels pointed slightly toward the direction of the move. ☐ ☐

Note: If possible, use a safety belt that has handles on the sides, because it is more comfortable for the person and provides less stress for you.

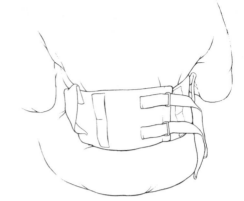

2. Tell the person that when you grasp the safety belt on the back side or by the handles, she must hold you around your shoulders. Grasp the safety belt on the back side of the person's waist, or by the handles, and have her hold you around your shoulders. ☐ ☐

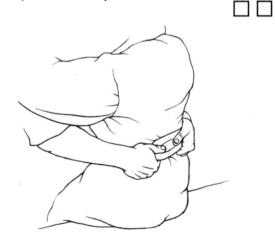

Note: Do not put pressure under the person's arms.

3. Place one foot facing the person with your knee (the one farther from the chair) between the person's knees and your other foot in the direction of the move. Flex your knees, tighten your abdominal and buttocks muscles, and keep your back straight. Put your head to the person's side closest to the chair so that you can keep the chair in sight during the move. ☐ ☐

4. Tell the person that on the count of three you are going to assist her to a standing position. Rock back and forth gently on each count to create momentum and, on the count of three, straighten your knees and pull her toward you. Remember to keep your back straight. ☐ ☐

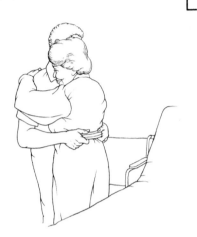

5. Shift your weight to the foot facing the direction of the move and turn so that she is right in front of the wheelchair. Ask her to tell you when she can feel the chair against the back of her legs. ☐ ☐

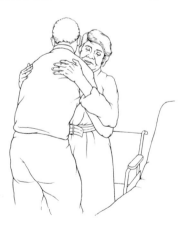

6. Lower the person into the wheel-chair by bending your knees and keeping your back straight. The person can help by placing her hands on the chair arms and help-ing to lower herself into the chair. ☐ ☐

7. Remove the safety belt. ☐ ☐

Option 3: Two Nurse Assistants Using a Safety Belt

Use this option if the person may be pre-dictable, but may not be consistent about helping to bear his own weight. If the per-son weighs over 125 lbs. and cannot sup-port his weight, use a mechanical lift. The caregiver must be able to get close enough to the person to avoid reaching.

1. Stand in front of the person, fac-ing him, and put the safety belt around his waist. The belt should be snug but not tight. The person should be sitting with his buttocks on the edge of the bed and his feet flat on the floor and his heels pointed slightly toward the direc-tion of the move. ☐ ☐

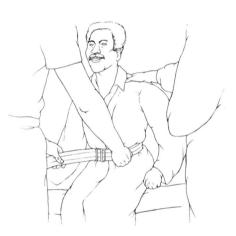

Note: If possible, use a safety belt that has handles on the sides, because it is more comfortable for the person and provides less stress for you.

2. Tell the person that you and your co-worker will grasp the safety belt on the back sides or on each handle and put an arm under each of his arms to move him into a standing position. ☐ ☐

3. Stand facing the person with your feet apart, with one foot pointing toward the person and the other foot pointing in the direction of the move. Flex your knees and keep your back straight. □ □

4. You and your co-worker grasp the safety belt on the back side or by the handles, with one hand, and you each put your free arm under one of his arms and hold onto his back. If you are using a walking belt, grasp the handles of the belt at his sides. □ □

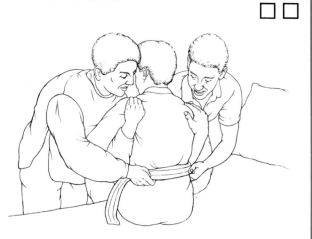

Note: Do not put pressure under the person's arms.

5. Tighten your abdominal and buttock muscles, flex your knees, and keep your back straight. □ □

6. Tell the person and your co-worker that on the count of three you are going to assist him to a standing position. On each count, gently rock back and forth to create momentum. On the count of three, pull the person toward you into a standing position by straightening your knees. □ □

7. Turn him until he is right in front of the wheelchair. Ask him to tell you when he can feel the wheelchair against the back of his legs. □ □

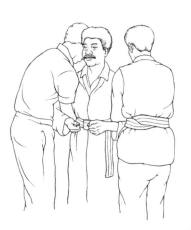

8. You and your co-worker each move to one side of the wheelchair and lower the person into the wheelchair, by bending your knees and keeping your back straight. The person can help by reaching back to hold onto the arm rests of the chair. □ □

9. Remove the safety belt. □ □

Completion

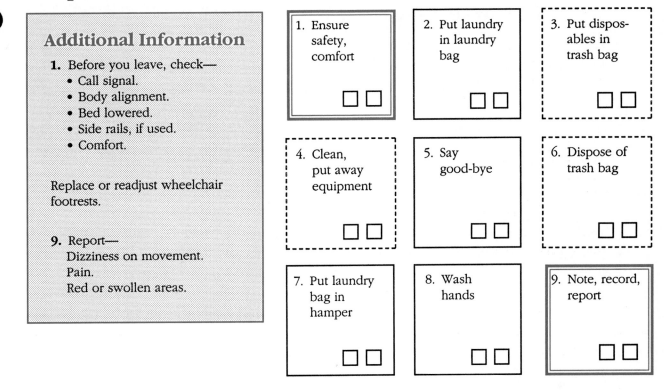

1. Ensure safety, comfort ☐ ☐

2. Put laundry in laundry bag ☐ ☐

3. Put disposables in trash bag ☐ ☐

4. Clean, put away equipment ☐ ☐

5. Say good-bye ☐ ☐

6. Dispose of trash bag ☐ ☐

7. Put laundry bag in hamper ☐ ☐

8. Wash hands ☐ ☐

9. Note, record, report ☐ ☐

_____

Student   Date

_____

Instructor   Date

Skill 19: Repositioning a Person in a Chair (2 Nurse Assistants)

Precautions

- Use proper body mechanics. To avoid injuring your back, always tighten your abdominal and buttock muscles when positioning someone.
- Make sure the wheelchair brakes are locked.
- Ask a co-worker to help you.
- Do not use a safety belt if the person has—
  - Had recent abdominal, chest, or back surgery.
  - Severe respiratory problems.
  - Severe cardiac problems.

Preparation

1. Gather supplies
  - Safety belt (if person is not already wearing one) ☐ ☐

Additional Information

4. Introduce your co-worker.

5. Explain your repositioning plan to the person and the co-worker. Tell them what they can do to help. Encourage the person to help as much as possible.

2. Focus ☐ ☐	3. Knock and wait ☐ ☐	4. Introduce and identify ☐ ☐
5. Explain ☐ ☐	6. Place supplies ☐ ☐	7. Wash hands ☐ ☐
8. Gather and prepare ☐ ☐	9. Adjust bed ☐ ☐	10. Provide privacy ☐ ☐

Notes:

Procedure

1. Lock the brakes of the person's wheelchair and put a safety belt on her, if she is not already wearing one. ☐ ☐

2. Stand as close as possible to the back of the wheelchair, facing the person's back. ☐ ☐

3. To give yourself a broad base of support, place one leg against the back of the wheelchair and put the foot of your other leg slightly behind and shoulder-width apart from the first leg. Bend your knees. ☐ ☐

4. Ask your co-worker to assist by kneeling on one knee close to the person's legs and placing an arm under her knees. ☐ ☐

5. Support the person's head against your chest or one shoulder, and grip the safety belt firmly with your palms up. Tighten your abdominal and buttock muscles, keep your back straight. ☐ ☐

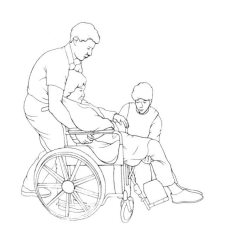

6. Tell the person and your co-worker that on the count of three you are going to move him back. ☐ ☐

7. On the count of three, your co-worker slightly lifts the person's legs and guides them toward the back of the chair, while you lift her by slowly straightening your legs. ☐ ☐

Note: Slide the person's legs and hips by transferring her weight toward the back of the chair at the same time you lift. Your co-worker must be careful not to twist her back.

Completion

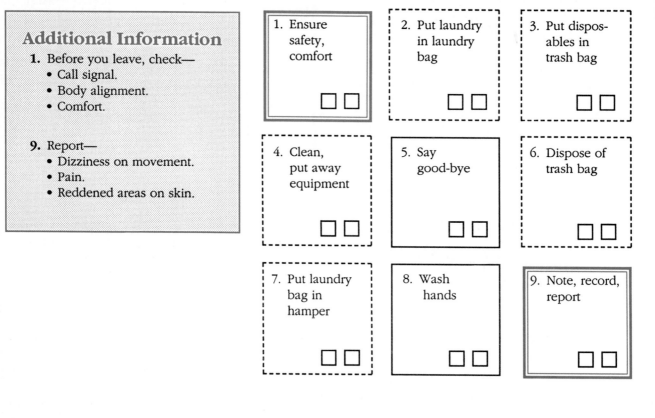

Additional Information

1. Before you leave, check—
   - Call signal.
   - Body alignment.
   - Comfort.

9. Report—
   - Dizziness on movement.
   - Pain.
   - Reddened areas on skin.

1. Ensure safety, comfort ☐ ☐

2. Put laundry in laundry bag ☐ ☐

3. Put disposables in trash bag ☐ ☐

4. Clean, put away equipment ☐ ☐

5. Say good-bye ☐ ☐

6. Dispose of trash bag ☐ ☐

7. Put laundry bag in hamper ☐ ☐

8. Wash hands ☐ ☐

9. Note, record, report ☐ ☐

_____

Student   Date

_____

Instructor   Date

Skill 20: Using a Mechanical Lift to Transfer a Person from the Bed to a Chair (2 Nurse Assistants)

Precautions

- Do not use a mechanical lift—
  - Until you have been properly instructed on how to use it and have practiced using it.
  - If parts are missing or broken.
- Assess the person and the room environment to determine your plan for moving him safely. Talk with your supervising nurse and check the care plan.
- Use proper body mechanics. To avoid injuring your back, always tighten your abdominal and buttocks muscles when positioning or transferring someone.
- Make sure bed brakes are locked.
- Ask a co-worker to help.

Note: For safety, two nurse assistants should always perform this transfer together. However, sometimes in a home setting you may have no choice except to operate the lift by yourself. Do not do this until you have the skill to do it.

Preparation

1. Gather supplies
   - Mechanical lift, which has the following parts:
   - Base, or frame
   - Sling—a canvas or plastic seat that extends from the back of the knees to the shoulder blades to provide support to the person being lifted
   - Chains or straps—used to attach the sling and suspend it from the base. On newer models, the sling may attach directly to hooks on the lift frame
   - Crank or handle—used to raise or lower the sling ☐ ☐

Additional Information

4. Introduce your co-worker.

5. Explain your transferring plan to the person and the co-worker. Tell them what they can do to help. Encourage the person to help as much as possible.

8. Gather the person's own—
   - Robe.
   - Slippers.
   - Wheelchair or straight chair.

9. Check for the placement of drainage tubes, and unhook or move them as necessary. Adjust the bed to a height that allows you to get the sling under the person and still maintain proper body mechanics.

2. Focus ☐ ☐

3. Knock and wait ☐ ☐

4. Introduce and identify ☐ ☐

5. Explain ☐ ☐

6. Place supplies ☐ ☐

7. Wash hands ☐ ☐

8. Gather and prepare ☐ ☐

9. Adjust bed ☐ ☐

10. Provide privacy ☐ ☐

Notes:

Procedure

1. Detach the sling from the metal hooks of the lift and fanfold half of it. ☐ ☐

2. Roll the person toward you and place the fanfolded part of the sling along her back, making sure it is smooth for comfort. Make sure the top of the sling is under her shoulders and the bottom end is at her knees. Roll her over the fanfolds, toward your co-worker, and onto the flat part of the sling. Straighten out the fanfolds. Help her lie flat. ☐ ☐

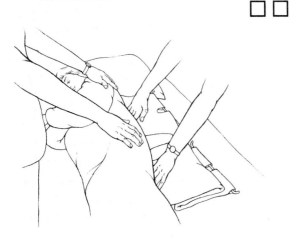

Note: You can help the person put on her bathrobe while she is turning from side to side. Make sure her clothing is wrinkle free. Put her slippers on at this time, too.

3. Wheel the lift into place over the person with the base beneath the bed. Make sure the bottom frame of the lift is in its widest position to provide a wide base of support during the move. Set the brakes on the lift. ☐ ☐

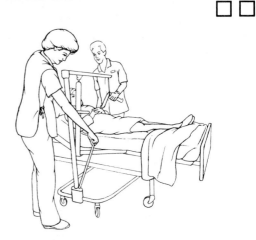

4. Attach the sling to the mechanical lift according to the manufacturer's instructions. Make sure the open ends of the **S**-shaped hooks face away from the person. ☐ ☐

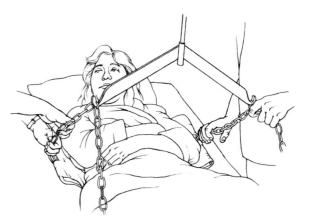

Why? The hooks can catch clothing or scrape skin if they are not facing the correct way.

5. Using the crank, slowly lift the person from the bed, release the brakes, and guide the lift away from the bed to the chair. Your co-worker guides the person's legs. Make sure the person is properly aligned and securely suspended. She may feel more secure if her arms are placed across her chest or if she can grasp the straps or chains. ☐ ☐

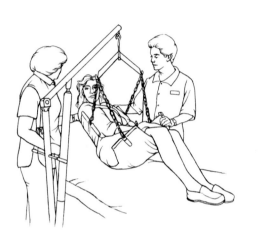

6. Set the brakes on the lift, and slowly lower the person into the chair and position her comfortably. Your co-worker should gently push on the person's knees while lowering her into the chair so that she moves into a sitting position in the chair. Your co-worker guides and steadies the person. ☐ ☐

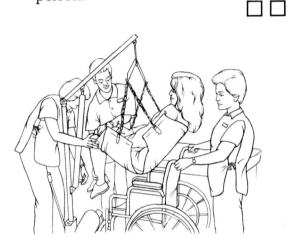

7. Remove the hooks from the frame of the lift and the sling. Keep the sling under the person, since you will later move her back to the bed. Make sure the fabric of the sling is wrinkle free. ☐ ☐

Completion

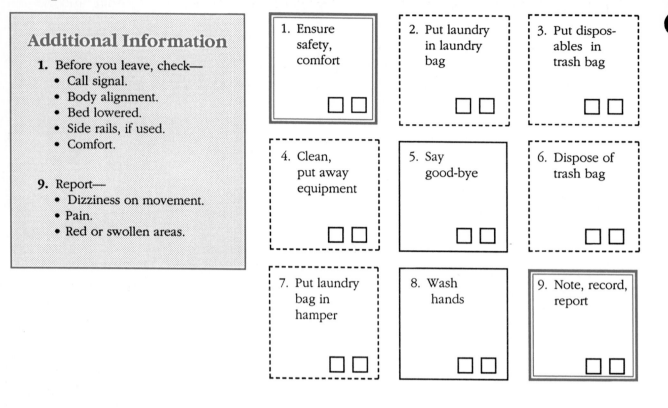

1. Ensure safety, comfort	2. Put laundry in laundry bag	3. Put disposables in trash bag
4. Clean, put away equipment	5. Say good-bye	6. Dispose of trash bag
7. Put laundry bag in hamper	8. Wash hands	9. Note, record, report

_____

Student   Date

_____

Instructor   Date

84

Skill 21: Brushing and Flossing a Person's Teeth

Precautions

- Slide (do not snap) the floss carefully between the teeth without pressing against the gums. Gums are soft, and dental floss can easily cut them.
- Always mix mouthwash with water. Gums are sensitive, and full-strength mouthwash may hurt them.
- Replace the person's toothbrush every 3 to 4 months or when it begins to fray or show wear. A worn toothbrush cannot properly clean the teeth and may injure the gums.
- Use a toothbrush with soft bristles. Also, use just enough pressure so that you get good contact with the tooth surface without flattening the bristles.

Preparation

1. Gather supplies
   - One towel
   - Two pairs of disposable gloves
   - Lip cream or petroleum jelly and cotton-tipped applicator
   - Plastic trash bag
   - Laundry bag (or plastic bag for wet or soiled linens)
   ☐ ☐

Additional Information

1. Bring a mask and protective eyewear if there is a likelihood that you will be splashed with bloody saliva, or if the person is HIV or HBV positive.

8. Gather the person's own —
- Emesis basin (small, kidney-shaped basin).
- Mouthwash.
- Drinking cup.
- Soft-bristled toothbrush with rounded or polished bristles.
- Fluoridated toothpaste.
- Dental floss.
- Petroleum jelly.

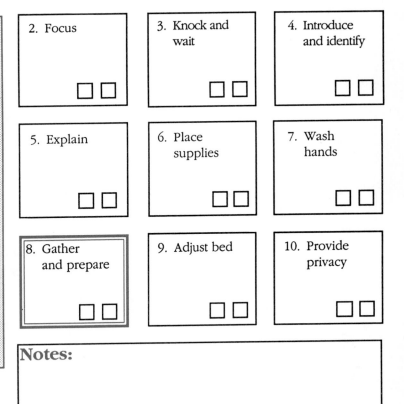

2. Focus ☐ ☐

3. Knock and wait ☐ ☐

4. Introduce and identify ☐ ☐

5. Explain ☐ ☐

6. Place supplies ☐ ☐

7. Wash hands ☐ ☐

8. Gather and prepare ☐ ☐

9. Adjust bed ☐ ☐

10. Provide privacy ☐ ☐

Notes:

Procedure

1. In a drinking cup, prepare a solution of half water and half mouthwash. ☐ ☐

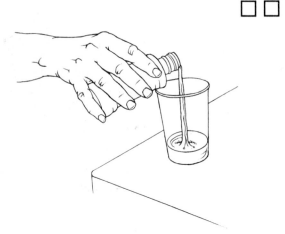

2. Lower the side rail, if used, on the side where you are working. ☐ ☐

3. Help the person turn her head toward you. ☐ ☐

Why? You can see better while you brush and floss.

4. Unfold the towel. Place it across the person's chest. ☐ ☐

5. Put on disposable gloves and any other necessary protective gear. ☐ ☐

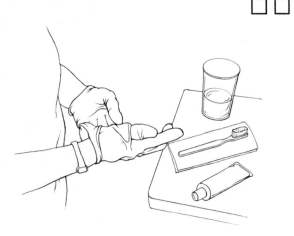

Why? Whenever you come in contact with mucous membranes that line the inside of the mouth, wear gloves to observe universal precautions.

6. Place the emesis basin on the towel under the person's chin. Ask her to hold it, if she is able. ☐ ☐

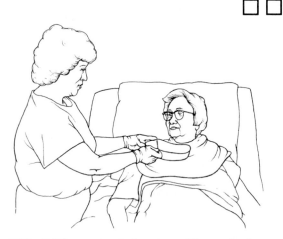

Why? The emesis basin will catch the brushing and rinsing liquids from the person's mouth.

7. Give the person a mouthful of the mouthwash mixture to rinse her mouth. Hold the emesis basin under her chin to catch the liquid. Wipe her chin, if necessary. ☐ ☐

Why? The mouthwash mixture moistens the person's mouth and gums, making it easier to brush his teeth.

8. Wet the toothbrush by holding it over the emesis basin and pouring mouthwash solution over it. ☐ ☐

Why? Toothpaste spreads more easily on a wet brush.

9. Put toothpaste on the wet brush. ☐ ☐

10. Clean the person's mouth by first brushing the upper teeth and gums:

- Place the toothbrush on the outer surface of the upper teeth at about a 45-degree angle.

- Move the brush back and forth, using very short strokes and a gentle scrubbing motion.

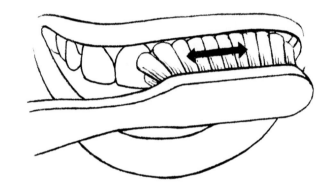

- Scrub the chewing surfaces of the upper teeth.

- Put the brush vertically against the inside surfaces of the front upper teeth and brush with a gentle up-and-down motion.

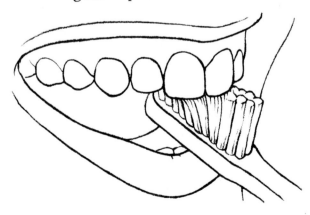

- Brush the lower teeth and gums in the same way, and brush the tongue very gently. ☐ ☐

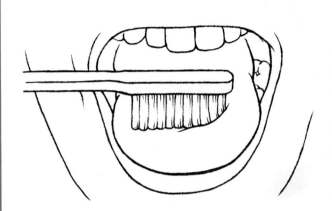

Why? Brushing the lower teeth first would produce too much spit, or saliva. Brushing the tongue helps control bacteria that can cause mouth odor.

11. Help the person rinse her mouth with the mouthwash mixture. Hold the emesis basin under her chin to catch the liquid. Wipe her chin, if necessary. ☐ ☐

12. To get the dental floss ready,—

- Break off about 18 inches of floss from the dispenser. (Measure it from the tip of your middle finger to your elbow.)

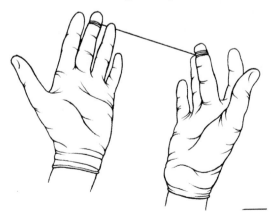

—

- Wrap most of the floss around the middle finger of one of your hands. Wrap the remaining floss around the middle finger of the other hand, leaving 1 inch of floss between your hands.

- Stretch it tightly between your thumbs and index fingers. □ □

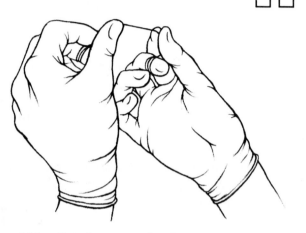

13. Gently insert the floss between each tooth without pressing against her gums. Use a gentle sawing motion to guide the floss between the teeth, never "snapping" it into the gums.

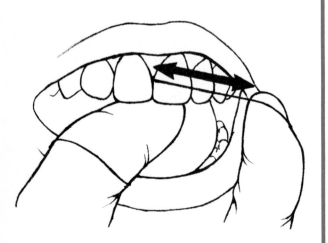

Hold the floss against the tooth and scrape the side of the tooth, moving the floss away from the gum. □ □

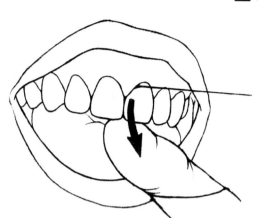

Why? Pressing or inserting the floss into the gum line can cause the gums to bleed. Gums also may bleed if the teeth have not been cleaned for a long time or if an infection is present.

After you floss each tooth, unwrap a clean 1-inch section of floss from your finger and wrap the soiled floss around the other finger.

Floss the teeth in this order: Start between the two front teeth, then do the first half of the upper teeth, the second half of upper teeth, the first half of lower teeth, the second half of the lower teeth.

Note: Remember to floss the back sides of the last teeth.

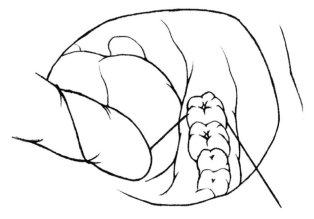

14. Place used floss in the plastic trash bag. ☐ ☐

15. Help the person rinse her mouth with the mouthwash mixture. Hold the emesis basin under her chin to catch the liquid. Wipe her chin, if necessary. ☐ ☐

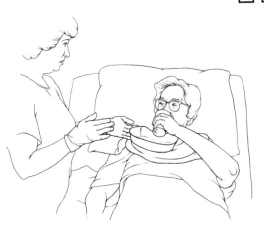

16. Remove disposable gloves and place them in the plastic trash bag. ☐ ☐

17. Raise the side rail, if used. ☐ ☐

Completion

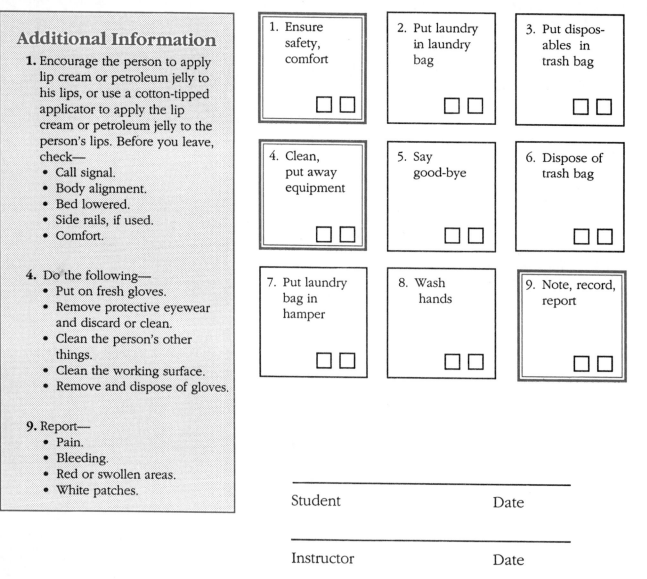

Additional Information

1. Encourage the person to apply lip cream or petroleum jelly to his lips, or use a cotton-tipped applicator to apply the lip cream or petroleum jelly to the person's lips. Before you leave, check—
- Call signal.
- Body alignment.
- Bed lowered.
- Side rails, if used.
- Comfort.

4. Do the following—
- Put on fresh gloves.
- Remove protective eyewear and discard or clean.
- Clean the person's other things.
- Clean the working surface.
- Remove and dispose of gloves.

9. Report—
- Pain.
- Bleeding.
- Red or swollen areas.
- White patches.

1. Ensure safety, comfort ☐ ☐

2. Put laundry in laundry bag ☐ ☐

3. Put disposables in trash bag ☐ ☐

4. Clean, put away equipment ☐ ☐

5. Say good-bye ☐ ☐

6. Dispose of trash bag ☐ ☐

7. Put laundry bag in hamper ☐ ☐

8. Wash hands ☐ ☐

9. Note, record, report ☐ ☐

Student _____ Date

Instructor _____ Date

Skill 22: Providing Denture Care

Precautions

- Dentures, or false teeth, are very expensive. You must handle them very carefully so that they do not get damaged. Dentures are very slippery when coated with mucus or saliva.
- Always mix mouthwash with water. Gums are sensitive, and full-strength mouthwash may hurt them.
- The person should remove his dentures for at least 8 hours every day to rest his gums.

Preparation

1. Gather supplies
   - One washcloth
   - One towel
   - Two pairs of disposable gloves
   - Tissues
   - Disposable mouth sponges
   - Lip cream or petroleum jelly and cotton-tipped applicator or gauze squares
   - Plastic trash bag
   - Laundry bag (or plastic bag for wet or soiled linens) ☐ ☐

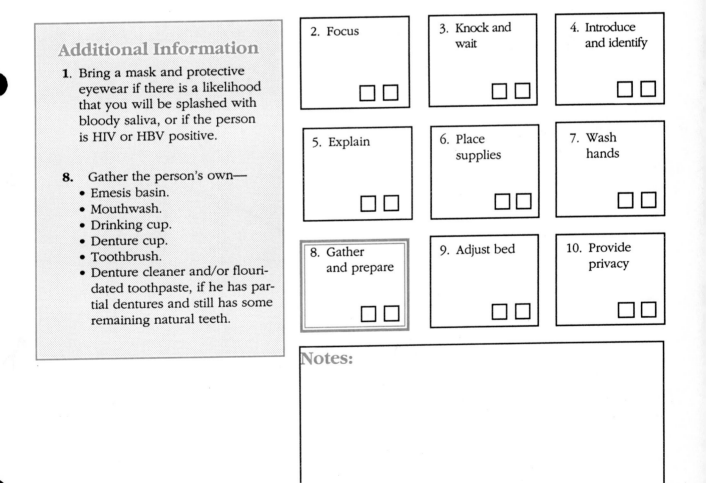

Additional Information

1. Bring a mask and protective eyewear if there is a likelihood that you will be splashed with bloody saliva, or if the person is HIV or HBV positive.

8. Gather the person's own—
   - Emesis basin.
   - Mouthwash.
   - Drinking cup.
   - Denture cup.
   - Toothbrush.
   - Denture cleaner and/or flouridated toothpaste, if he has partial dentures and still has some remaining natural teeth.

2. Focus ☐ ☐

3. Knock and wait ☐ ☐

4. Introduce and identify ☐ ☐

5. Explain ☐ ☐

6. Place supplies ☐ ☐

7. Wash hands ☐ ☐

8. Gather and prepare ☐ ☐

9. Adjust bed ☐ ☐

10. Provide privacy ☐ ☐

Notes:

Procedure

The tasks for denture care are—
1. Removing dentures.
2. Providing care for the person's mouth.
3. Cleaning and replacing dentures.

Task 1: Removing Dentures

1. In a drinking cup, prepare a solution of half water and half mouthwash. ☐ ☐

2. Lower the side rail, if used, on the side where you are working. ☐ ☐

3. Ask the person to turn his head toward you. ☐ ☐

4. Unfold the towel. Place it across the person's chest. ☐ ☐

5. Put on disposable gloves and any other necessary protective gear. ☐ ☐

6. Place the emesis basin on the towel under the person's chest. Ask him to hold it, if he is able. ☐ ☐

7. Ask the person to rinse his mouth with the mouthwash mixture. Hold the emesis basin to catch the liquid. Wipe his chin, if necessary. ☐ ☐

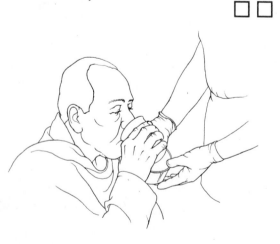

Why? Dentures are easier to remove if the mouth is moist.

8. Ask the person to remove his dentures and put them in the denture cup. ☐ ☐

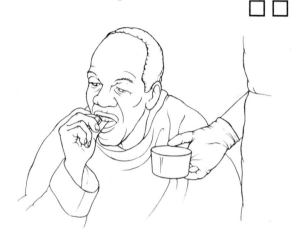

If he needs assistance, use a tissue to hold his teeth firmly with your thumb and index finger.

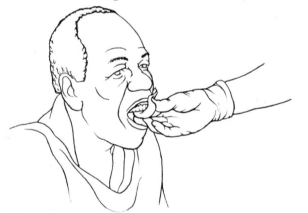

Then, with a rocking motion, gently remove the teeth and put them in the denture cup.

Why? If you use a rocking motion when removing dentures, it breaks the seal that holds the dentures in place.

9. Put the denture cup on the overbed table or nightstand. Check the identification mark on the dentures to make sure that the name matches the person. ☐ ☐

Task 2: Providing Care for the Person's Mouth

1. Give the person a mouthful of the mouthwash mixture to rinse his mouth. Hold the emesis basin under his chin to catch the liquid. Wipe his chin, if necessary. ☐ ☐

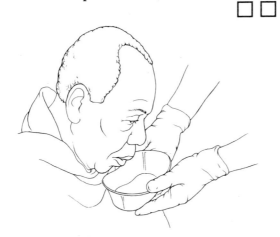

2. Help the person clean his mouth with mouth sponges dipped in mouthwash mixture. ☐ ☐

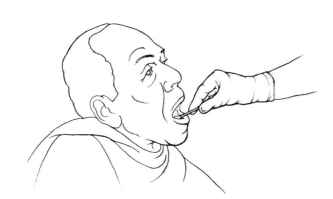

If he has any of his natural teeth, help him clean them, using the toothbrush and fluoridated toothpaste, and floss them.

Help him clean his entire mouth:
- Roof
- Tongue
- Inside of cheeks
- Gums
- Under tongue
- Lips

Change the mouth sponges when they become coated with mucus, or gummy saliva. Put the used mouth sponges in the plastic trash bag. ☐ ☐

3. Help the person rinse his mouth with the mouthwash mixture. Hold the emesis basin under his chin to catch the liquid. Wipe his chin, if necessary. ☐ ☐

4. Raise the side rail, if used, and lower the bed. ☐ ☐

Task 3: Cleaning and Replacing Dentures

1. Take the denture cup, toothbrush, toothpaste, washcloth, and towel to the sink. ☐ ☐

2. Line the sink with the washcloth. ☐ ☐

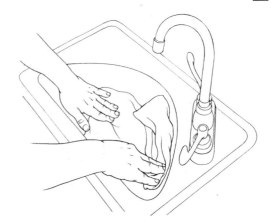

Why? Lining the sink with a washcloth keeps the dentures from chipping or breaking if they fall while you are cleaning them.

3. Turn on the faucet with a fresh paper towel. Adjust the water temperature so that it is cool. ☐ ☐

Why? Cool water is safer for the dentures. Hot water may change the shape, or warp, the dentures.

4. Wet the toothbrush. ☐ ☐

5. Put toothpaste on the wet brush. ☐ ☐

6. Allow the sink to fill half full with cool water. Use the paper towel to turn off the faucet. ☐ ☐

7. Remove the dentures from the cup and hold them over the sink. Use the toothbrush to clean them. Brush all surfaces. ☐ ☐

8. Rinse the dentures under cool, running water. ☐ ☐

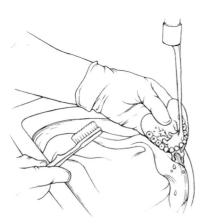

9. Hold the dentures in one hand. Rinse the denture cup with the other hand and put the clean dentures back in the denture cup. Use a paper towel to turn the faucet on and off. ☐ ☐

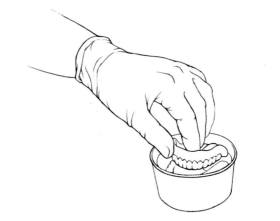

10. Help the person put the dentures back in his mouth. If he prefers not to wear the dentures now, leave the clean dentures in the denture cup and add with enough water to cover them. ☐ ☐

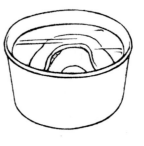

Why? If dentures are covered with water in the denture cup, they won't become dry and warped.

Note: Do not soak dentures overnight in denture cleaner because it may weaken the metal parts.

11. Remove disposable gloves and place them in a plastic trash bag. ☐ ☐

12. Raise the side rail, if used. ☐ ☐

Completion

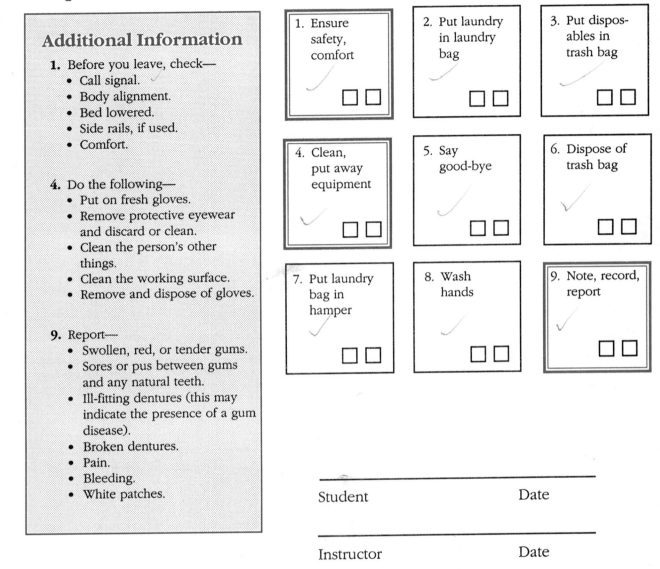

Additional Information

1. Before you leave, check—
- Call signal.
- Body alignment.
- Bed lowered.
- Side rails, if used.
- Comfort.

4. Do the following—
- Put on fresh gloves.
- Remove protective eyewear and discard or clean.
- Clean the person's other things.
- Clean the working surface.
- Remove and dispose of gloves.

9. Report—
- Swollen, red, or tender gums.
- Sores or pus between gums and any natural teeth.
- Ill-fitting dentures (this may indicate the presence of a gum disease).
- Broken dentures.
- Pain.
- Bleeding.
- White patches.

1. Ensure safety, comfort

2. Put laundry in laundry bag

3. Put disposables in trash bag

4. Clean, put away equipment

5. Say good-bye

6. Dispose of trash bag

7. Put laundry bag in hamper

8. Wash hands

9. Note, record, report

_____

Student   Date

_____

Instructor   Date

Skill 23: Providing Mouth Care for an Unconscious Person

Precautions

- When working on an unconscious person, open the mouth gently, without using force.
- Always position the person's head to the side so that he won't aspirate, or breathe in, any fluids into the lungs. An unconscious person cannot swallow fluids.
- Always mix mouthwash with water. Gums are sensitive, and full-strength mouthwash may hurt them.
- Use a toothbrush with soft bristles. Use just enough pressure to give you good contact with the tooth surface without flatening the bristles.

Preparation

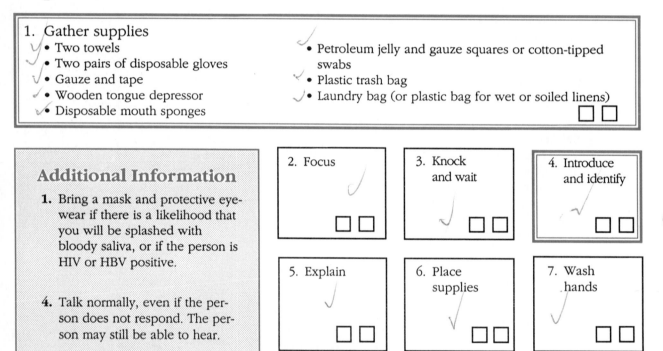

1. Gather supplies
   - Two towels
   - Two pairs of disposable gloves
   - Gauze and tape
   - Wooden tongue depressor
   - Disposable mouth sponges
   - Petroleum jelly and gauze squares or cotton-tipped swabs
   - Plastic trash bag
   - Laundry bag (or plastic bag for wet or soiled linens) ☐ ☐

Additional Information

1. Bring a mask and protective eyewear if there is a likelihood that you will be splashed with bloody saliva, or if the person is HIV or HBV positive.

4. Talk normally, even if the person does not respond. The person may still be able to hear.

8. Gather the person's own—
   - Emesis basin.
   - Mouthwash.
   - Drinking cup.
   - Soft-bristled toothbrush with rounded or polished bristles.

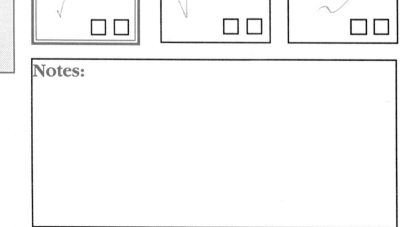

2. Focus ☐ ☐

3. Knock and wait ☐ ☐

4. Introduce and identify ☐ ☐

5. Explain ☐ ☐

6. Place supplies ☐ ☐

7. Wash hands ☐ ☐

8. Gather and prepare ☐ ☐

9. Adjust bed ☐ ☐

10. Provide privacy ☐ ☐

Notes:

Procedure

1. Make a padded tongue depressor by placing one or two tongue blades together and wrapping gauze squares around one end. Use tape to hold it securely. ☐ ☐

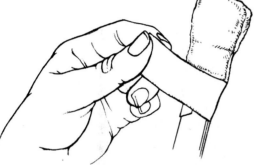

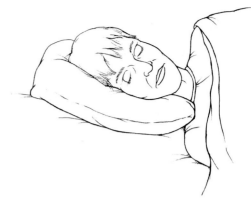

6. Unfold one towel. Gently lift her head and spread the towel under it. ☐ ☐

Why? The towel protects her pillow.

7. Unfold the second towel. Place it across the person's chest. ☐ ☐

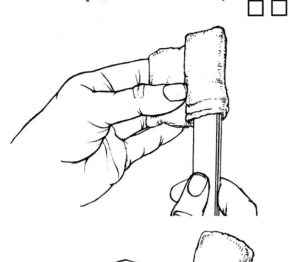

2. In a drinking cup, prepare a solution of half water and half mouthwash. ☐ ☐

3. Lower the side rail, if used, on the side of the bed where you are working. ☐ ☐

4. Position the person on her side with her face extended over the edge of the pillow. ☐ ☐

5. Turn her head toward you. ☐ ☐

8. Place the emesis basin on the towel near the person's cheek. ☐ ☐

9. Put on disposable gloves. ☐ ☐

10. Without using force, gently separate the person's upper and lower teeth. To do this, cross the middle finger and thumb of one hand. Put the thumb against the person's top teeth, and the other against the person's lower teeth and gently push the finger and thumb apart. This causes her jaw to open.

Use the padded tongue depressor as a prop to hold her mouth open. ☐ ☐

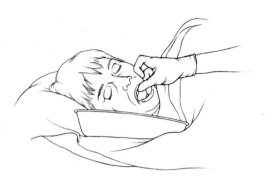

Change the mouth sponges when they become coated with mucus. Put the used mouth sponges in the plastic trash bag. If there is a great deal of thick mucus or secretions, wrap gauze squares around your finger to remove them. ☐ ☐

12. Use a soft toothbrush moistened with diluted mouthwash to clean his teeth. Be careful not to use too much fluid so that the person does not aspirate. ☐ ☐

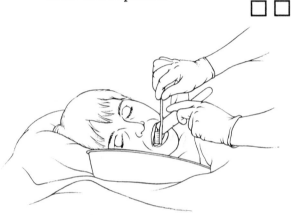

11. Clean the soft tissues of the person's mouth with a mouth sponge dipped in diluted mouthwash. Use just enough fluid to moisten the sponge. ☐ ☐

Clean his entire mouth:
- Roof
- Inside of cheeks
- Teeth
- Gums
- Under tongue
- Lips

13. Apply a small amount of petroleum jelly to the person's lips, using a cotton swab or gauze square. ☐ ☐

14. Remove the gloves and throw them away in the plastic trash bag. ☐ ☐

15. Raise the side rail, if used. ☐ ☐

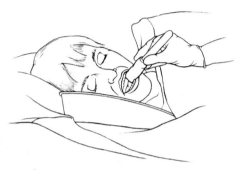

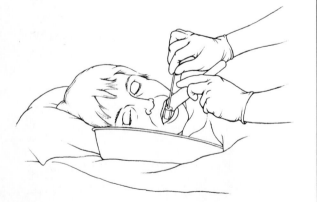

Completion

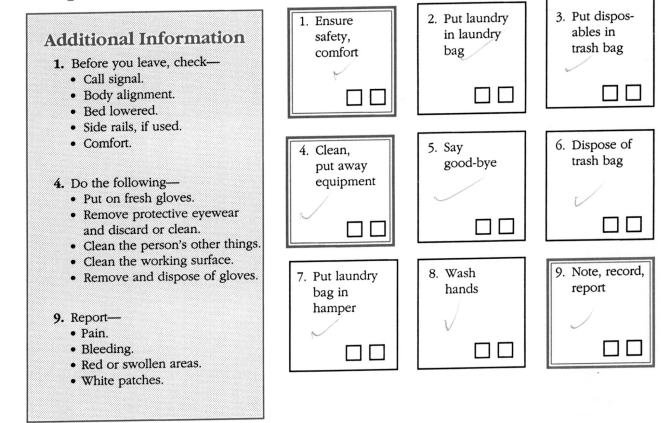

Additional Information

1. Before you leave, check—
- Call signal.
- Body alignment.
- Bed lowered.
- Side rails, if used.
- Comfort.

4. Do the following—
- Put on fresh gloves.
- Remove protective eyewear and discard or clean.
- Clean the person's other things.
- Clean the working surface.
- Remove and dispose of gloves.

9. Report—
- Pain.
- Bleeding.
- Red or swollen areas.
- White patches.

1. Ensure safety, comfort

2. Put laundry in laundry bag

3. Put disposables in trash bag

4. Clean, put away equipment

5. Say good-bye

6. Dispose of trash bag

7. Put laundry bag in hamper

8. Wash hands

9. Note, record, report

Student   Date

_____

Instructor   Date

Skill 24: Giving a Person a Complete Bed Bath and Shampoo

Precautions

- Keep the person well covered to provide privacy and warmth.
- Check the water temperature. It should be warm to the touch on the inside of your wrist. If the water is too hot, it can injure the person's skin. If the water is too cold, it can chill the person.
- Use proper body mechanics as you wash the person and move him from back to side.
- Inspect the person's skin for injuries, changes in condition and color (such as reddened areas or bruises), and sores.
- Wash the perineal area of a female from front to back. This decreases infection.
- When giving a shampoo, cover the person's eyes with a washcloth to prevent shampoo from getting into his eyes.
- Check for placement of drainage tubes, and unhook or move them, as necessary.
- Ask a co-worker to help, if needed.

Preparation

1. Gather supplies.

For the bath:
- Bath blanket (a flannel sheet used to keep the person warm during bathing)
- Three towels
- Two washcloths
- Disposable bed protector
- Disposable gloves
- Plastic trash bag
- Laundry bag (or plastic bag for wet or soiled linens)

For the shampoo:
- Two towels
- Two washcloths
- Waterproof chair
- Waterproof sheet
- Shampoo tray, plastic sheet, or large plastic trash bag
- Cup or pitcher (for rinsing the hair)
- Empty washbasin

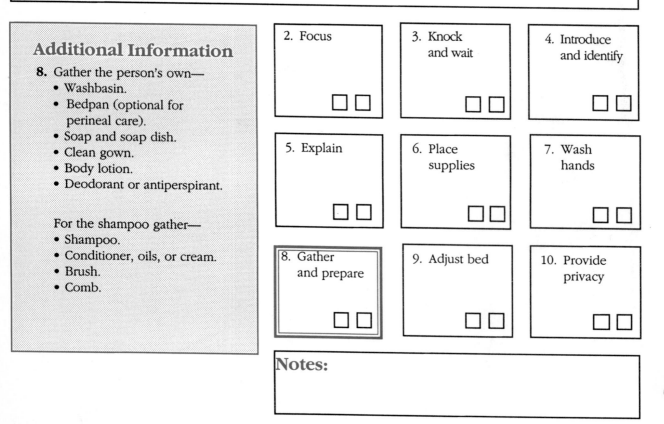

Additional Information

8. Gather the person's own—
- Washbasin.
- Bedpan (optional for perineal care).
- Soap and soap dish.
- Clean gown.
- Body lotion.
- Deodorant or antiperspirant.

For the shampoo gather—
- Shampoo.
- Conditioner, oils, or cream.
- Brush.
- Comb.

2. Focus

3. Knock and wait

4. Introduce and identify

5. Explain

6. Place supplies

7. Wash hands

8. Gather and prepare

9. Adjust bed

10. Provide privacy

Notes:

Procedure

The tasks for giving a complete bed bath are—

1. Bathing the person.
2. Rubbing the person's back.
3. Cleaning the person's perineal area.
4. Shampooing the person's hair (optional).

Task 1: Bathing the Person

1. Fill the washbasin with warm water and place it on the overbed table. Check the temperature of the water. □ □

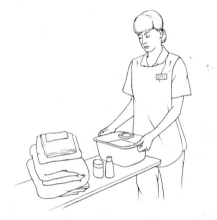

Note: If the person has very dry skin, add a few drops of bath oil or olive oil if the person can tolerate it, to the bath water to help seal in moisture.

2. Adjust the angle of the head of the bed to a flat position. If the person has difficulty breathing when lying flat, lower the head as much as possible. Make sure the person is comfortable and breathing easily. □ □

Why? Putting the person in this position prevents you from injuring your back and makes it easier for the person to turn onto his side.

3. Lower the side rail, if used, on the side where you are working. Help the person move closer to the side of the bed where you are working. □ □

4. Remove and fold the bedspread and blanket for re-use. Put the bath blanket over the person.

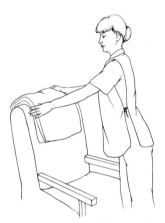

Why? The bath blanket protects the person's privacy while you undress and bathe him. It also keeps him from becoming chilled.

Have the person hold the bath blanket under his chin. If the person can't hold the blanket, tuck the edges of the blanket under the person's shoulders or pillow while you roll the top sheet down. Place your hand under the bath blanket and roll the top sheet to the bottom of the bed. □ □

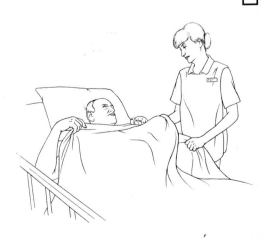

Note: If you are going to change the bed linens following the bath, remove the top sheet and put it in the laundry bag at the foot of the bed. Otherwise, roll it down to the foot of the bed, but do not remove it.

5. Take off the person's gown by slipping it off each arm and pulling it from under the bath blanket on the side closest to you.

☐ ☐

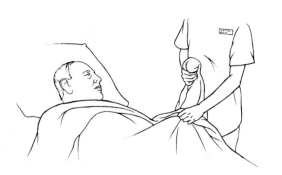

Why? When you remove the gown beneath the blanket, the person stays warm. Also, his body isn't exposed.

6. Unfold the towel. Place it across the person's chest.

☐ ☐

Why? The towel protects the bath blanket while you wash his face.

7. Wet the washcloth and make a mitt with it by—
   • Holding a corner of the washcloth between your thumb and fingers.

☐ ☐

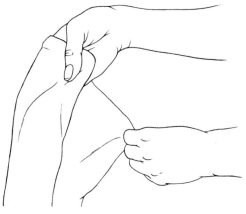

   • Wrapping the rest of the cloth around your hand and holding it with your thumb.

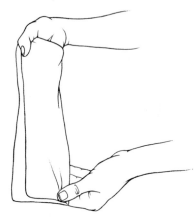

   • Folding the cloth over your fingers and tucking it under the fold in your palm.

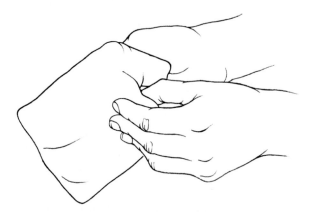

Why? Making a mitt prevents the edge of the washcloth from dragging over the person's skin, which causes chilling.

8. Without using soap, use the washcloth to bathe the eye farthest from you. Always begin at the inner corner of the eye, near the nose. Then move the washcloth across the eye to the outer corner. Use the towel to dry the eye. Use the opposite end of the mitt and towel to bathe and dry the other eye. □ □

Note: Ask the person if he wants you to use soap on his face.

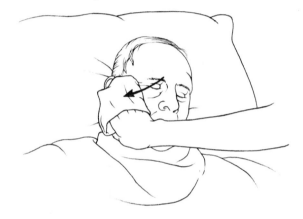

Why? Using opposite ends of the washcloth and towel to wash and dry each eye prevents the spread of germs from one eye to the other.

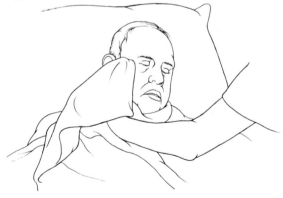

9. Wash, rinse, and dry the person's face, neck, and ears. Be sure to wash and dry behind the ears. Use soap sparingly. □ □

10. Fold back the bath blanket on the person's arm that is farther from you. Place the towel lengthwise under his arm. Wash, rinse, and dry his shoulder, arm, and underarm, or axilla. Use the towel that was under the arm to dry it. □ □

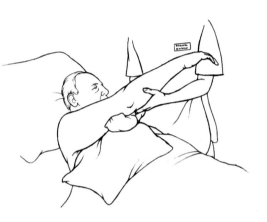

Why? If you begin with the arm farther away, you won't drip water on the arm you have already cleaned and dried. Remember to support the joints as you hold the person's arm.

Note: Remember, if the bed is not elevated, work on one side of the person at a time. This prevents you from bending and reaching, which could hurt your back.

Note: If the person wants to use a deodorant or antiperspirant, apply it at this time or wait until after the bath.

11. Wash, rinse, and dry the person's hand. When possible, place his hand in the washbasin. To do this, place a bed protector on the bed. Place the basin on top of the bed protector, and place the person's hand in the basin or place the basin on the overbed table. ☐ ☐

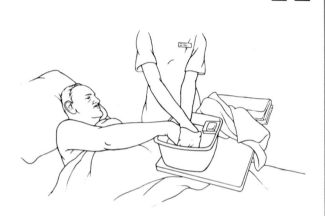

Why? Soaking the person's hand promotes thorough cleaning and loosens dirt under his nails.

Remove the towel from under his arm, and cover it with the bath blanket.

12. Fold back the bath blanket on the person's arm that is nearer to you. Place the towel lengthwise under his arm. Wash, rinse, and dry his shoulder, arm, axilla, and hand.

Remove the towel from under his arm, and cover it with the bath blanket. Place the towel over person's chest and abdomen on top of the bath blanket. ☐ ☐

13. Reach under the towel that is over the bath blanket and fold the bath blanket down to the person's pubic area without exposing it. Leave the towel in place so that the person is not completely exposed. ☐ ☐

14. Fold back the towel to expose the side of the person's chest that is farther from you. Wash, rinse, and dry the person's chest. ☐ ☐

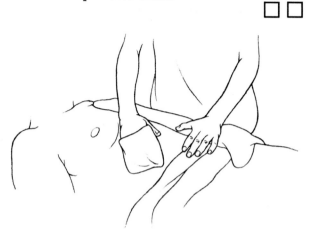

Inspect under the person's breast and skin folds as you work. Dry his skin completely. Re-cover his chest with the towel.

Why? Moisture in skin folds can result in skin cracking. Later, these cracks can lead to skin irritation or sores. If the person can tolerate it, use talcum powder sparingly between skin folds to reduce moisture. Make sure his skin is dry before applying powder.

15. Fold back the towel to expose the side of the person's chest that is nearer to you. Wash, rinse, and dry his chest. ☐ ☐

16. Wash, rinse, and dry the person's stomach, or abdomen, in the same manner as the chest, doing the farther side first, then the nearer side.

Pull the bath blanket back up to cover his chest and abdomen, and remove the towel from underneath. ☐ ☐

17. Check to make sure the water is still warm. Also check to make sure the water has not become too soapy. If the water is too cool or has become too soapy,—
   * Raise the side rail, if used.
   * Empty and rinse the washbasin.
   * Refill the washbasin with warm water.
   * Check the temperature of the water.
   * Return to the bed and lower the side rail, if used. ☐ ☐

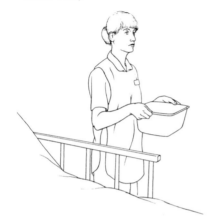

18. Fold the bath blanket away from the person's leg that is farther from you. Place the towel lengthwise under his leg. Wash his leg and foot. When possible, place his foot in the washbasin. To do this, move the towel down under the foot. Move the washbasin onto the towel. Help the person bend his knee and place his foot into the washbasin. ☐ ☐

Why? Soaking the person's foot promotes thorough cleaning and loosens dirt under his toenails.

Use the mitt to wash the person's foot.

Rinse his leg and foot. Help him move his leg out of the washbasin and onto the towel. Move the washbasin back to the overbed table or nightstand. Use the towel to dry his leg and foot, making sure the skin between his toes is dry. Re-cover his leg with the bath blanket. Remove the towel from under his leg.

19. Fold the bath blanket away from the person's leg that is nearer to you. Place the towel under his leg. Wash, rinse, and dry his leg and foot. When possible, place his foot in the washbasin. Re-cover his leg with the bath blanket. Remove the towel from under his leg. ☐ ☐

20. Help the person turn onto one side so that his back is facing you. (Use the procedure you learned in Skill 13, Moving a Person Around in Bed.) □ □

21. Place the towel on the sheet behind the person's neck, back, and buttocks. Drape the bath sheet over the person's chest, shoulders, abdomen, and legs. Wash, rinse, and dry the person's neck, back, and buttocks. Inspect the skin as you work. □ □

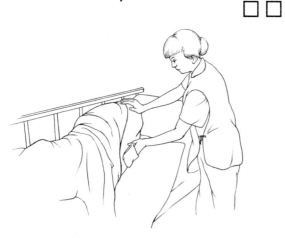

Task 2: Rubbing the Person's Back

1. Squeeze some lotion onto the palm of your hand. □ □

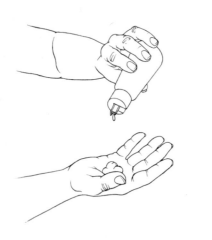

Warm it by rubbing your hands together. Do not squeeze lotion directly onto the person's skin. □ □

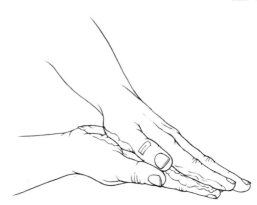

2. Gently rub the person's back. Use big circular motions. Start at the base of his back and move upward toward his shoulders. Without stopping the motion or taking your hands away, rub his back, moving downward toward his buttocks. □ □

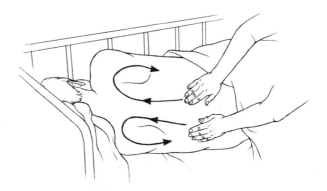

Why? When you move your hands from the base of the spine toward the shoulders, it promotes comfort. It also stimulates circulation toward the heart. If you keep moving with even, continuous strokes, it relaxes and comforts the person.

Continue the backrub for 3 to 5 minutes.

3. If you are doing the backrub as part of the person's bed bath and will be going on to bathe his perineal area, place a bed protector on the bed under his buttocks and roll him onto his back. If you are doing the backrub separately from the bed bath, roll the person onto his back and go on to the completion steps. ☐ ☐

4. Raise the side rail, if used. ☐ ☐

5. Empty the water from the washbasin into the sink. Wash out the washbasin. ☐ ☐

Task 3: Cleaning the Person's Perineal Area

1. Fill the washbasin with warm water. ☐ ☐

2. Check the temperature of the water. ☐ ☐

3. Place a bed protector under the person's hips. ☐ ☐

4. If the person is able to do his or her own perineal care, offer a fresh washcloth, soap, and clean water. Give him or her a few minutes alone to bathe. ☐ ☐

5. If the person is unable to do his or her own perineal care, use the following steps:

Perineal care for females

1. Drape the woman's perineal area by—

- Placing the bath blanket over her like a diamond. Put one corner at her neck, a corner at each side, and one corner between her legs.

- Helping her bend her knees and spread her legs.

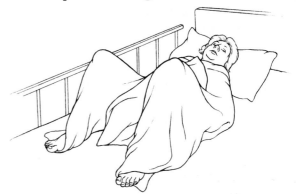

- Wrapping each side corner around her feet. Do this by bringing each side corner under and around a foot, then over the top, and finally by tucking the corner under her foot. This keeps the blanket from sliding off of her. ☐ ☐

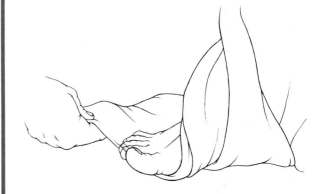

2. Elevate her pelvis by placing either a bedpan or a folded towel (or bath blanket) under her buttocks. ☐ ☐

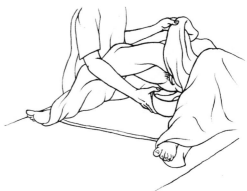

Why? This position raises the hips, or pelvis, which gives you a better view of her perineal area. The folded towel or bedpan collects excess water during care.

3. Put on disposable gloves for infection control. ☐ ☐

4. Make the washcloth into a mitt. ☐ ☐

5. Lift the corner of the bath blanket between her legs, and fold it back onto her abdomen to expose her perineal area. ☐ ☐

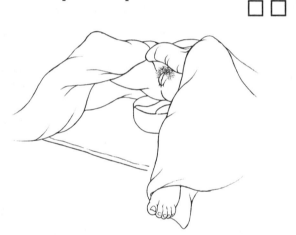

6. Put soap on the mitt and wash her perineal area with the soapy washcloth by—
   • Washing the pubic hair on her lower abdomen.

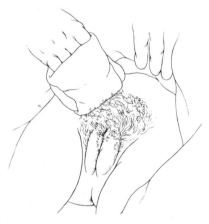

• Separating her labia with one hand.
• Washing one side of her labia in one gentle, even stroke, then the other side. Move in the direction from her hair, or pubic area, to her anal area.
• Washing gently down the middle. Move in the direction from her pubic area to her anal area.

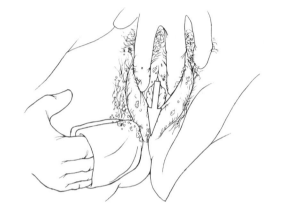

Why? Washing from front to back decreases contamination of the urethral opening with bacteria from the anal opening.

Use a different area of the washcloth for each stroke. ☐ ☐

Why? Using an unused section of the washcloth prevents the spread of germs.

7. Rinse the soap out of the washcloth. Rinse her perineal area by using the same steps as you did when washing. ☐ ☐

8. Dry her perineal area with a clean towel, using the same steps as you did when washing and rinsing. ☐ ☐

9. Remove the bedpan or the folded towel or blanket. ☐ ☐

10. Assist the person as she rolls onto her side. ☐ ☐

11. Wash and rinse her anal area. Work in the direction away from the genital area. Use a different area of the washcloth for each stroke. ☐ ☐

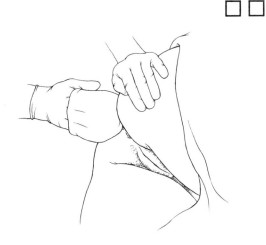

12. Dry her anal area thoroughly. ☐ ☐

Why? Moisture may cause skin irritation and sores.

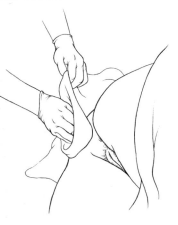

13. Take off the gloves and throw them away in the plastic trash bag. ☐ ☐

14. Roll the bed protector up against the woman's back, and help her roll onto her back and then onto her side so that she is facing you. Raise the side rail, if used. Go to the opposite side of the bed, lower the side rail, if used, and remove the bed protector and put it in the plastic trash bag. Assist the person as she rolls onto her back, and cover her with the bath blanket. Raise the side rail, if used. ☐ ☐

15. Empty the water from the washbasin into the sink and wash the washbasin. ☐ ☐

16. Wash your hands. ☐ ☐

Perineal care for males

1. Adjust the bath blanket over the man like a diamond. Put one corner at his neck, a corner at each side, and one corner between his legs. ☐ ☐

2. Put on disposable gloves for infection control. ☐ ☐

3. Make the washcloth into a mitt. ☐ ☐

4. Lift the corner of the bath blanket between the man's legs and fold it back to expose the perineal area. ☐ ☐

5. Put soap on the mitt. Hold the man's penis in one hand. Retract the foreskin if he is uncircumcised. Wash the tip of his penis with the soapy washcloth. Always wash from the urethral opening outward, using a circular motion. ☐ ☐

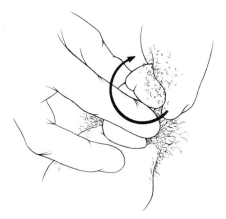

Why? Washing in this direction helps prevent contamination of the urethral opening.

Use a different area of the washcloth for each stroke.

Why? Using an unused section of the washcloth prevents the spread of germs.

6. Rinse the soap from the washcloth. Rinse and pat dry the tip of his penis, using the same steps as you did when washing. If the man is uncircumcised, return the foreskin to its natural position. ☐ ☐

7. Wash, rinse, and pat dry the shaft of his penis. Always work toward the pubic area. ☐ ☐

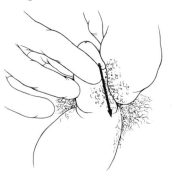

8. Assist the man as he spreads his legs under. Wash, rinse and pat dry his scrotum and surrounding area thoroughly.

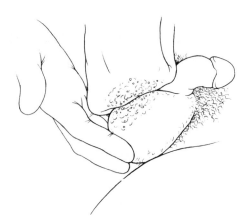

9. Assist him to roll onto his side. ☐ ☐

10. Wash, rinse, and pat dry his anal area. Use a different area of the washcloth for each stroke. ☐ ☐

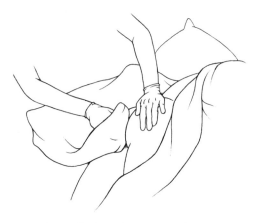

11. Take off the gloves and throw them away in the plastic trash bag. ☐ ☐

12. Roll the bed protector up against the man's back, and help him roll onto his back and then onto his side so that he is facing you. Raise the side rail, if used. Go to the opposite side of the bed, lower the side rail, if used, and remove the bed protector and put it in the plastic trash bag. Assist the man as he rolls onto his back, and cover him with the bath blanket. Raise the side rail, if used. ☐ ☐

13. Empty the water from the washbasin into the sink and wash the washbasin. ☐ ☐

14. Wash your hands. ☐ ☐

Task 4: Shampooing the Person's Hair

1. With the person either sitting up or lying down, remove any pins or clips from the hair. Brush or comb the hair to remove any tangles. ☐ ☐

2. Place the waterproof chair on the side of the bed where you are working. Move it close to the head of the bed. ☐ ☐

3. Fill the washbasin with warm water. Check the temperature of the water. Place the washbasin on a clean surface. ☐ ☐

4. Place an empty washbasin on the chair. ☐ ☐

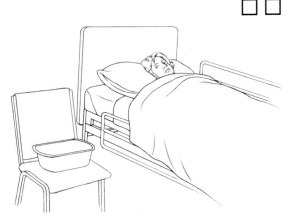

Note: If you are shampooing separately from a complete bed bath, lower the head of the bed to a flat position, if possible. If the person is unable to lie flat, lower the head of the bed as much as possible. Make sure the person is comfortable and breathing easily. Replace the top sheet with the bath blanket as you would for a bed bath. ☐ ☐

5. Lower the side rail, if used, on the side where you are working. ☐ ☐

6. Place a waterproof sheet under the person's head so that it covers the bottom sheet. ☐ ☐

Why? The waterproof sheet keeps the bedding from getting wet.

7. Place the shampoo tray under the person's head so that the drainage through it is directed toward the empty washbasin on the chair. ☐ ☐

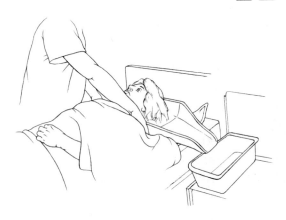

If you are using a plastic sheet or large trash bag, place a rolled towel inside the bag. Twist it into a **C** shape. Place the person's head in the center of the **C**. Drape the sheet or bag toward the side of the bed so that water drains into the washbasin on the chair. ☐ ☐

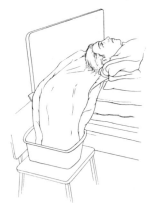

8. Place a clean washcloth over the person's eyes. ☐ ☐

9. Fill the cup with (clean) water from the washbasin. Wet her hair. Continue filling the cup and wetting her hair until it is fully wet. ☐ ☐

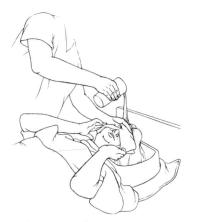

10. Apply a small amount of shampoo to her hair, and use both hands to wash it. Massage her scalp gently with your fingertips until it is completely lathered. Start at the hairline and work toward the back of her head. ☐ ☐

11. Fill the cup with water from the washbasin. Rinse the person's hair. Continue filling the cup and rinsing her hair until all the shampoo is removed. ☐ ☐

12. If the person wishes, wash and rinse her hair again, just as you did in the previous steps. ☐ ☐

13. If the person wants to use conditioner on her hair, apply it now. Work it through with your fingertips. ☐ ☐

14. Fill the cup with water and rinse her hair until the conditioner is removed. ☐ ☐

15. Unfold a clean, dry towel. Gently lift the person's head and towel dry by rubbing the hair with the towel. If the person seems chilled, wrap her head in the towel. ☐ ☐

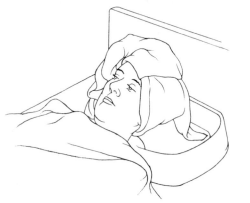

16. Remove the shampoo tray and plastic sheet or large trash bag from beneath the person's head, as well as the waterproof sheet. Place the reusable equipment on the chair. Throw away any disposable supplies in the plastic trash bag. ☐ ☐

Note: After the person is dressed, help her brush and comb her hair. Style it the way the person likes it. (You will learn how to help brush and comb in Skill 27.)

Note: Make sure the person's hair is dry before she goes to bed or goes outside. Follow your supervising nurse's instructions on whether or not to use a portable hair dryer.

17. Help the person put on a clean gown or get dressed for the day. (You will learn how to help a person get dressed in Skill 33.)

18. Replace and straighten the top linens, or make the bed with fresh linens. (You will learn how to make an occupied bed in Skill 36.)

Completion

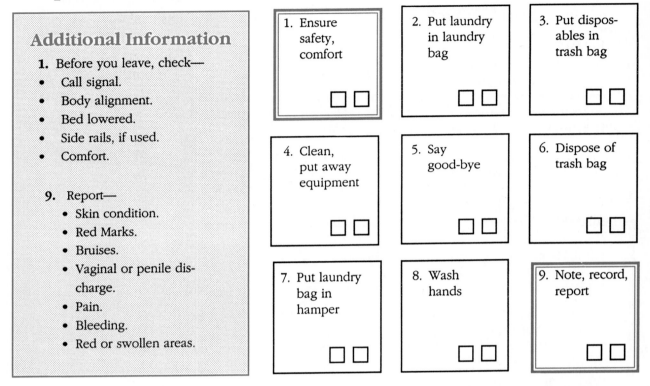

1. Ensure safety, comfort ☐ ☐

2. Put laundry in laundry bag ☐ ☐

3. Put disposables in trash bag ☐ ☐

4. Clean, put away equipment ☐ ☐

5. Say good-bye ☐ ☐

6. Dispose of trash bag ☐ ☐

7. Put laundry bag in hamper ☐ ☐

8. Wash hands ☐ ☐

9. Note, record, report ☐ ☐

_____
Student   Date

_____
Instructor   Date

Skill 25: Helping a Person with Showering and Shampooing

Precautions

- Make sure the person is well covered with a bathrobe and wears slippers when you take him to the shower room or bathroom to provide privacy and warmth.
- Check the water temperature. It should feel warm to the touch on the inside of your wrist. If the water is too hot, it can injure the person's skin. If the water is too cold, it can chill the person.
- Inspect the person's skin for injuries, changes in condition and color (such as reddened areas or bruises), and sores.
- When giving a shampoo, cover the person's eyes with a washcloth to prevent shampoo from getting into them.
- To prevent injury, always stay with the person.

Preparation

1. Gather supplies
   - Bath blanket (a flannel sheet used to keep the person warm after bathing or showering)
   - Two towels (three towels if the person is going to shampoo)
   - One washcloth
   - Shower cap (if not shampooing)
   - Disposable gloves, if you need to help the person with perineal care
   - Plastic trash bag
   - Laundry bag (or plastic bag for wet or soiled linens)
   - Wheelchair (if person does not have her own) or shower chair, if needed
   - Plastic apron (optional)

Additional Information

1. Reserve the shower room (if you are assisting someone in a hospital or nursing home).
   - Make sure the shower is clean and the room is warm.
   - Assess the person to determine if he can walk or will need to ride in a wheelchair or shower chair.
   - Determine the need for a shower chair or shower seat.

Note: If a person in unsteady on his feet, he may need to sit down during the shower. A shower chair is a waterproof chair on wheels that can be used to move a person into and out of the shower. A shower seat is a removable chair or bench in the shower for a person to sit on while in the shower. If you use one of these, clean the seat with disinfectant cleaner.

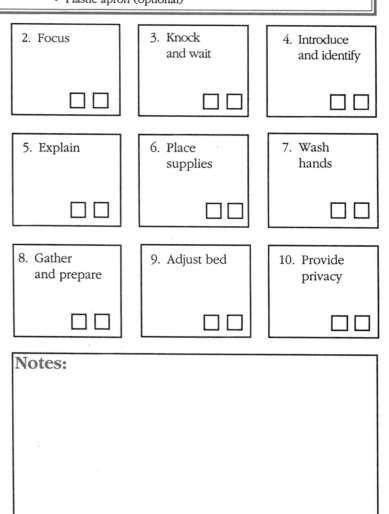

2. Focus

3. Knock and wait

4. Introduce and identify

5. Explain

6. Place supplies

7. Wash hands

8. Gather and prepare

9. Adjust bed

10. Provide privacy

Notes:

Procedure

1. Help the person undress. Help him put on her bathrobe and slippers. (The soles of the slippers should be nonskid to prevent falls.) ☐ ☐

2. Accompany the person to the shower room or bathroom, helping him as necessary. If he is using a wheelchair or shower chair, have him hold the supplies in his lap. ☐ ☐

Why? The person should be supervised during transportation so that he doesn't fall.

3. Turn the water faucet on, and adjust the temperature of the water so that it is warm to the touch on the inside of your wrist. ☐ ☐

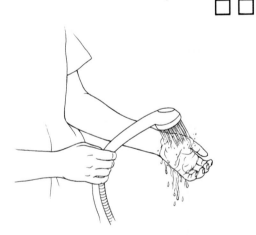

4. Help the person take off his bathrobe and slippers. ☐ ☐

Note: Some people need to sit down while removing their slippers. Provide a stable place to sit, such as a chair. Put a towel on the seat to provide comfort and help control infection.

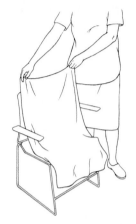

5. Put his bathrobe and slippers in a clean, dry place. ☐ ☐

6. If the person does not want to shampoo his hair, offer him a shower cap to keep his hair dry. ☐ ☐

7. Help him into the shower. If he uses a shower chair, be sure to lock the brakes or place the chair against the shower wall so that it does not slip. ☐ ☐

8. If the person is going to wash his own hair, give him any assistance he needs and skip to step 10. ☐ ☐

9. If he needs you to wash his hair, continue with the following steps.
   • Put on a plastic apron, if desired.
   • Give the person a clean washcloth to hold over his eyes. ☐ ☐

Why? The washcloth keeps shampoo, conditioner, and water from getting into his eyes.

- Wet his hair thoroughly. Redirect the spray nozzle as necessary to avoid getting yourself wet.

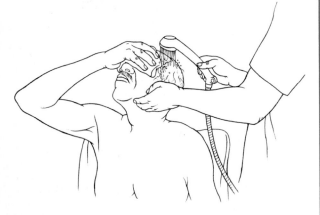

- Apply a small amount of shampoo on the person's hair. Use both hands to wash his hair. Massage his scalp gently with your fingertips until his hair is completely lathered. Be careful not to scratch his scalp with your fingernails.
- Rinse the shampoo out of his hair.
- If the person desires, shampoo and rinse again.
- If the person wants conditioner, apply it to his hair. Work it through with your fingertips.

Why? Conditioner takes tangles out of the hair, which makes it easier to comb and style.

- Rinse the conditioner out of his hair.

10. Give the person the soap. Encourage him to wash himself as much as possible. Assist him when he needs your help. If the person is unable to wash his perineal area, put on gloves and help him with this final washing step.

□ □

11. Make sure all soap is rinsed off his skin.

□ □

Why? Soap dries the skin. When you help the person rinse, inspect his skin for injuries or changes in condition.

12. Help the person get out of the shower and have him sit on the towel-covered chair.

□ □

Note: Call for a co-worker to help you, if needed. With some shower chairs on wheels, the person can be dried off and remain seated in the shower seat until returning to his own room.

13. Wrap the bath blanket around his shoulders for warmth and privacy.

□ □

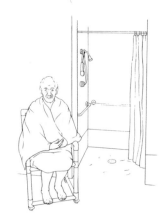

14. Shut off the water. ☐ ☐

15. Unfold the second towel and use it to towel dry the person's hair. Use this towel to wrap his head.

16. Unfold the third towel. Help the person dry off by patting gently with the towel. Make sure the areas between his toes and at all skin folds are completely dry. ☐ ☐

Why? Patting gently won't damage the skin as rubbing does. When you help the person dry off, inspect his skin for injuries or changes in condition. ☐ ☐

17. Help the person as he puts on his slippers. ☐ ☐

18. Help him as he stands up to put on his bathrobe. ☐ ☐

19. Put the wet towels and washcloths in the plastic laundry bag. ☐ ☐

20. If the person can walk without assistance, carry his personal things with you to the room as you escort him. Otherwise, first help him to the room, make sure he is safe, and go back to the shower room to get his things. If he uses a wheelchair to go back to his room, have him hold his things in his lap. ☐ ☐

Why? It is important to take care of the person's needs first.

21. If the person is able to tolerate it, apply lotion to his dry skin areas. ☐ ☐

22. Help him get dressed and comb his hair if needed. ☐ ☐

Note: Make sure the person's hair is dry. Follow your supervising nurse's instructions on whether to use a portable hair dryer.

Completion

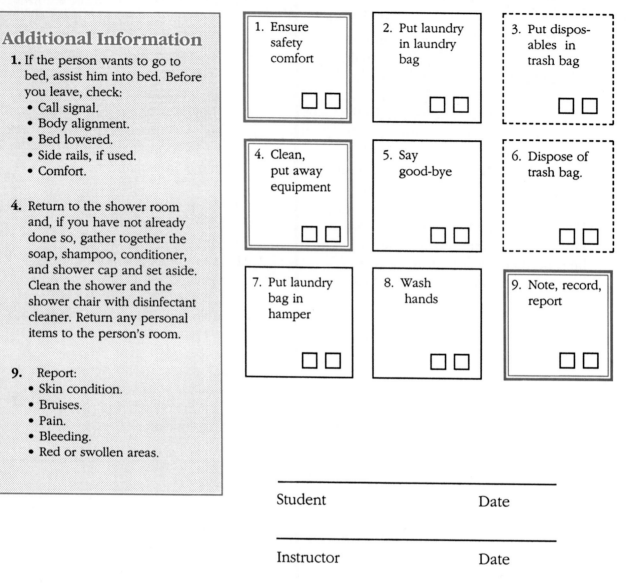

1. Ensure safety comfort ☐ ☐	2. Put laundry in laundry bag ☐ ☐	3. Put disposables in trash bag ☐ ☐
4. Clean, put away equipment ☐ ☐	5. Say good-bye ☐ ☐	6. Dispose of trash bag. ☐ ☐
7. Put laundry bag in hamper ☐ ☐	8. Wash hands ☐ ☐	9. Note, record, report ☐ ☐

Student _____ Date

Instructor _____ Date

Skill 26: Helping a Person with Bathing and Shampooing in the Tub

Precautions

- Make sure the person is well covered with a bathrobe and wears slippers when you take him to the tub to provide privacy and warmth.
- Check the water temperature with a bath thermometer. It should not be higher than 105° Fahrenheit. If the water is too hot, it can injure the person's skin. If the water is too cold, it can make the person chilled. If possible, ask the person if the water feels okay. Sometimes even water at 105° Fahrenheit will feel too warm for a person.
- Shut off the hot water faucet first. This prevents hot water from dripping from the faucet, which could scald the person.
- Be sure to use proper body mechanics when you help the person into and out of the tub.
- Inspect the person's skin for injuries, changes in condition and color (such as discoloration or bruises), and sores.

Preparation

1. Gather equipment and supplies.
   - Bath blanket
   - Bath thermometer
   - Two towels (three towels if he is going to shampoo)
   - Pitcher
   - One washcloth (two washcloths if he is going to shampoo)
   - Laundry bag (or plastic bag for wet of soiled linens)

   ☐ ☐

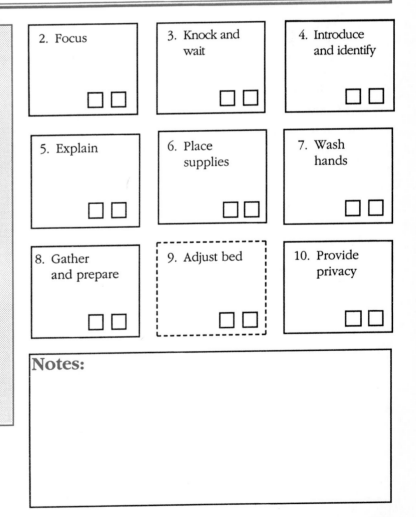

Additional Information

1. Reserve the tub room (if you are assisting someone in a hospital or nursing home).
   - Make sure the tub is clean, a nonskid bath mat is in the bottom of the tub, and the room is warm.
   - Assess the person to determine the best way to transport him to the tub room or bathroom and to help him in and out of the tub.

   Note: The person may walk or need to ride in a wheelchair. If the person is transported in a wheelchair, you may have to remove the stationary chair from the tub room or bathroom to make room to maneuver in the bathroom.

2. Focus ☐ ☐

3. Knock and wait ☐ ☐

4. Introduce and identify ☐ ☐

5. Explain ☐ ☐

6. Place supplies ☐ ☐

7. Wash hands ☐ ☐

8. Gather and prepare ☐ ☐

9. Adjust bed ☐ ☐

10. Provide privacy ☐ ☐

Notes:

Procedure

1. Help the person undress. Help her put on her bathrobe and slippers with nonskid soles. □ □

2. Accompany the person to the tub room or bathroom, helping her as necessary. If she is using a wheelchair, have her hold the supplies in her lap. Otherwise, first take the supplies to the tub room. Then return to the person's room to help her to the tub room. □ □

3. Ask her to sit in the chair next to the tub while you draw the bath water. □ □

4. Run water into the tub, filling it half way before turning off the hot water, then the cold. □ □

Use the bath thermometer to check the temperature. It should be 105° F. Add more hot water if the temperature is less than 105° F. Add more cold water if the temperature is more than 105° F.

Call for assistance if you need help getting the person into the tub.

5. As the person sits in the chair, help her take off her slippers. □ □

6. Help her stand up from the chair to take off her bathrobe. □ □

7. When helping her into the tub, use a broad base of support so that you can keep your balance. Keep the person close to you. Keep your back straight. Do not twist. Ask the person to lift one leg up and into the tub while you support and balance her. Then direct her to lift the other leg and bring it into the tub. Assist the person to sit down in the tub. □ □

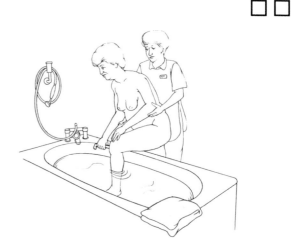

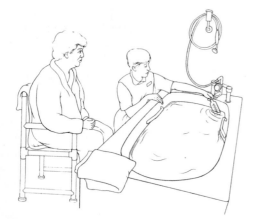

Why? Proper body mechanics help you and the person. They keep you from hurting yourself. They help you move the person safely from one place to another. Some specialty tubs have mechanical lifts that you can use to lift a person in and out of a tub. If you will be using one where you work, be sure to get special instruction and practice before you use it to assist a person.

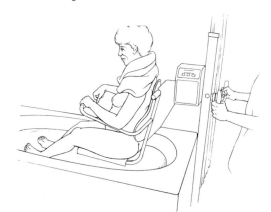

8. Put the person's bathrobe and slippers in a clean, dry place. ☐ ☐

9. Place a folded towel on the chair. ☐ ☐

10. If the person seems chilled, offer her a towel to throw over her shoulders as she bathes. ☐ ☐

11. Give the person the washcloth and soap. Encourage her to wash herself as much as possible, and remind her to use soap sparingly. Assist her when she needs your help. Let water out of the tub to lower the water level and put on gloves if you need to assist with cleaning her perineal area. Do this step last. ☐ ☐

12. Make sure all the soap is rinsed off her skin. ☐ ☐

13. If the person is going to wash her own hair, give her any assistance she needs and skip to step 15. If she needs you to wash her hair, continue with the following steps:
   - Give her a clean washcloth to hold over her eyes.
   - Wet her hair thoroughly.
   - Apply a small amount of shampoo to the person's hair. Use both hands to wash her hair. Massage her scalp gently with your fingertips until her hair is completely lathered. Be careful not to scratch her scalp.
   - Use the pitcher to pour water over the person's head to rinse the shampoo out of her hair.

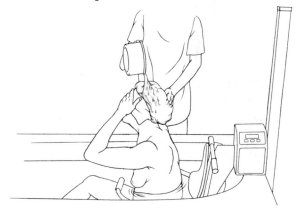

   - If the person desires, shampoo and rinse again.
   - If the person wants conditioner, apply it to her hair. Work it through with your fingertips.
   - Rinse the conditioner out of her hair. ☐ ☐

14. Unfold a towel and use it to towel dry the person's hair. Use this towel to wrap her head. ☐ ☐

15. Call for assistance if you need it to help the person out of the tub and help her as she sits on the towel-covered chair. Wrap the bath blanket around her. ☐ ☐

16. Unfold the second towel. Help the person with drying off by patting gently with the towel. Make sure the areas between her toes are completely dry. ☐ ☐

17. Help the person as she puts on her slippers. ☐ ☐

18. Help the person as she stands up to put on her bathrobe. ☐ ☐

19. Put the wet towels and washcloths in the plastic laundry bag. ☐ ☐

20. If the person can walk without assistance, carry her personal things back with you to the room as you escort her. Otherwise, first escort her to the room, and then go back to the tub room to get her things. If she uses a wheelchair to go back to her room, have her hold her things in her lap. ☐ ☐

21. Apply lotion to the person's dry skin areas. ☐ ☐

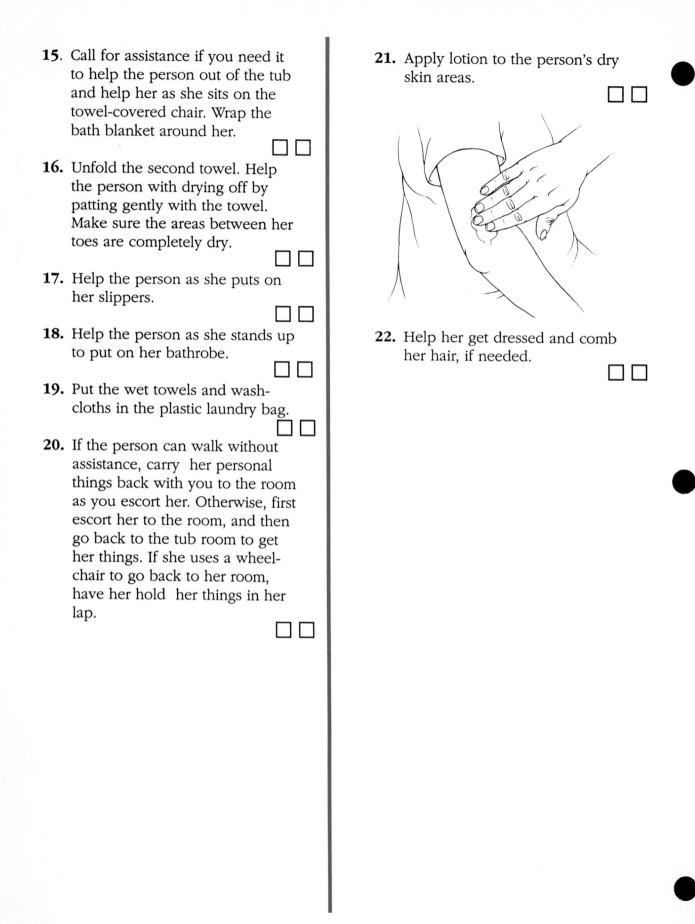

22. Help her get dressed and comb her hair, if needed. ☐ ☐

Completion

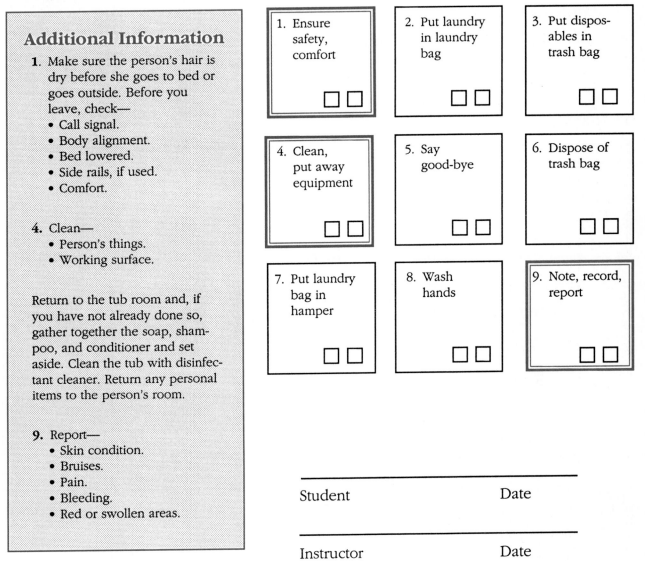

1. Ensure safety, comfort	2. Put laundry in laundry bag	3. Put disposables in trash bag
4. Clean, put away equipment	5. Say good-bye	6. Dispose of trash bag
7. Put laundry bag in hamper	8. Wash hands	9. Note, record, report

Student _____ Date _____

Instructor _____ Date _____

123

Skill 27: Brushing and Combing a Person's Hair

Precautions

- Brush and comb hair gently so that you do not pull out her hair.
- Use a brush or a comb with blunt teeth so that you won't hurt the person's scalp.

Preparation

1. Gather supplies
   - Towel
   - Laundry bag ☐ ☐

Additional Information

1. Remember to always wash your hands before gathering clean linens.

8. Gather the person's own—
   - Brush.
   - Comb.
   - Wide-tooth comb (if the person has tangles).
   - Hand mirror (if the person wants to look).

   Place the person's things on the clean surface.

9. It is easier to comb a person's hair when she is sitting, but you also can comb a person's hair when she is lying in bed. To do this, turn her head first to one side and then the other. Remember to adjust the height of the bed so that you do not have to bend and reach.

2. Focus ☐ ☐

3. Knock and wait ☐ ☐

4. Introduce and identify ☐ ☐

5. Explain ☐ ☐

6. Place supplies ☐ ☐

7. Wash hands ☐ ☐

8. Gather and prepare ☐ ☐

9. Adjust bed ☐ ☐

10. Provide privacy ☐ ☐

Notes:

Procedure

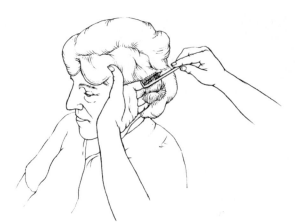

1. Place the towel over the person's shoulders. ☐ ☐

Why? Covering the shoulders with a towel prevents hair from falling onto the person's clothing.

Note: If the person is lying in bed, place the towel under her shoulders.

2. Remove the person's eyeglasses or any hair pins that she is wearing. ☐ ☐

3. Brush her hair gently and slowly. ☐ ☐

Why? Brushing hair gently keeps it from becoming damaged. It also stimulates circulation.

4. Start brushing gently at the ends of the hair, not at the scalp. Work your way up in sections to the scalp. Brush strokes should go away from the scalp. ☐ ☐

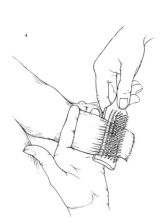

Why? This prevents the hair from breaking and detangles the ends.

Note: If the person's hair is tangled, a wide-tooth comb is easier to use than a narrow-tooth comb. Work slowly and in small sections. Forcing and pulling on a tangled mass breaks many hairs.

In extreme cases, wetting the hair and applying a conditioner and then combing the hair may help.

Why? Conditioner makes the hair slippery and easier to detangle. Wash and rinse hair after it is detangled.

5. Style the person's hair the way she likes it. ☐ ☐

Note: Remember, each person should decide how her hair is styled.

6. Encourage the person to see her hair as it is being styled. Offer to let her look in the hand mirror. ☐ ☐

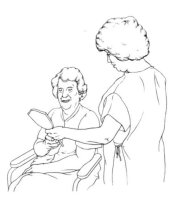

7. Remove the towel from the person's shoulders (or from beneath the head and shoulders) and put it in the laundry bag. ☐ ☐

8. If the person is going to stay in bed, raise the side rail, if used. ☐ ☐

Completion

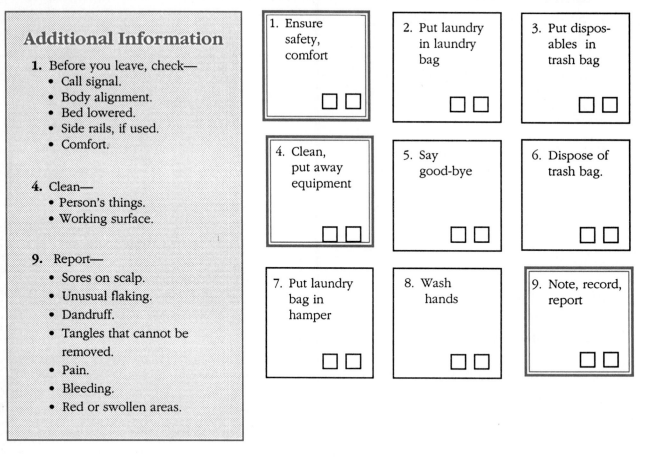

Additional Information

1. Before you leave, check—
- Call signal.
- Body alignment.
- Bed lowered.
- Side rails, if used.
- Comfort.

4. Clean—
- Person's things.
- Working surface.

9. Report—
- Sores on scalp.
- Unusual flaking.
- Dandruff.
- Tangles that cannot be removed.
- Pain.
- Bleeding.
- Red or swollen areas.

1. Ensure safety, comfort

2. Put laundry in laundry bag

3. Put disposables in trash bag

4. Clean, put away equipment

5. Say good-bye

6. Dispose of trash bag.

7. Put laundry bag in hamper

8. Wash hands

9. Note, record, report

_____

Student   Date

_____

Instructor   Date

Skill 28: Helping a Man Shave with a Safety Razor

Precautions

- Always ask your supervising nurse if a person should be shaved. Some medicines can cause excessive bleeding if a person is cut.
- Make sure each razor is used by only one person. Because blood particles may be left on the blade, sharing a razor may spread blood-borne infections.

Preparation

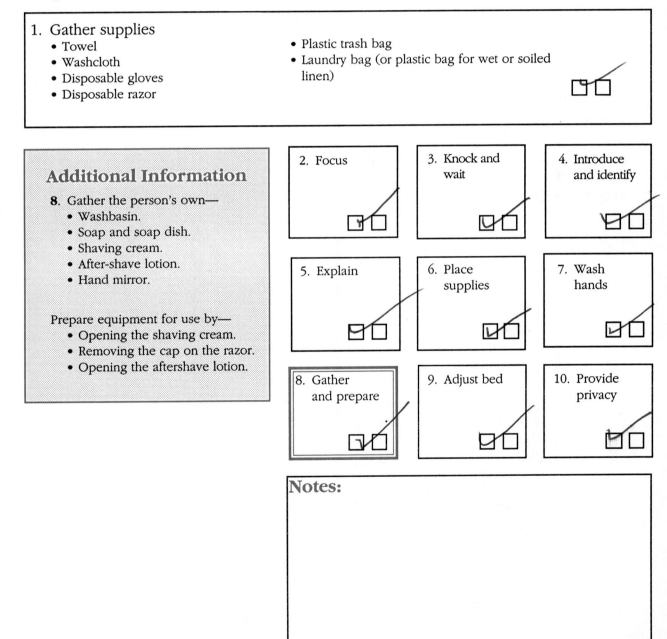

1. Gather supplies
   - Towel
   - Washcloth
   - Disposable gloves
   - Disposable razor
   - Plastic trash bag
   - Laundry bag (or plastic bag for wet or soiled linen)

Additional Information

8. Gather the person's own—
   - Washbasin.
   - Soap and soap dish.
   - Shaving cream.
   - After-shave lotion.
   - Hand mirror.

Prepare equipment for use by—
   - Opening the shaving cream.
   - Removing the cap on the razor.
   - Opening the aftershave lotion.

2. Focus

3. Knock and wait

4. Introduce and identify

5. Explain

6. Place supplies

7. Wash hands

8. Gather and prepare

9. Adjust bed

10. Provide privacy

Notes:

Procedure

1. Fill the washbasin with warm water. Use a paper towel to turn the faucet on and off. Place the basin on the clean surface.

Check the temperature of the water of see if it is warm to the touch on the inside of your wrist. ☑☐

2. Lower the side rail, if used, on the side of the bed where you are working. ☐☐

3. Help the person into a sitting position. ☑☐

Note: If the person is unconscious, elevate his head slightly.

4. Place the towel over his chest. ☑☐

Why? The towel protects the person's clothing.

5. Inspect his skin for moles, birthmarks, or sores. ☑☐

Why? You must shave carefully around these areas, because scraping or cutting can cause bleeding.

6. Using the washbasin of warm water, help the person wash his face. Use soap, if he prefers, and remove the soap with the wet washcloth. ☑☐

Why? Washing the face removes oil and bacteria from the skin. It also helps to raise the hair shafts so that they are easier to shave off.

7. Help the person as he puts shaving cream on his face. ☑☐

Why? Using shaving cream softens the skin and helps the razor glide over the skin, which prevents nicking and cutting.

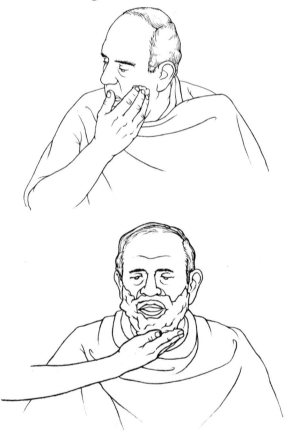

8. If you help the person shave, put on disposable gloves. ☑☐

Why? If bleeding occurs while you help the person shave, the gloves protect you from possible infection.

9. With the fingers of one hand, hold the person's skin tight as you use the razor to shave downward. By shaving downward, you are shaving in the direction that his hair grows. ☑☐

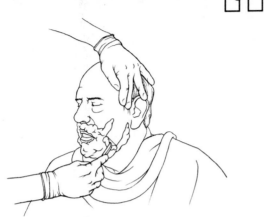

Why? Shaving in the direction that the hair grows produces a smoother shave. It also prevents the skin from becoming irritated.

10. Rinse the razor often in the washbasin of water to remove hair. ☑☐

Why? By rinsing the razor often, the cutting edge remains clean.

11. Use shorter strokes around the person's chin and lips. Work downward toward his neck under his chin. Shave one side of the face first and then the other. ☑☐

12. Use the wet washcloth to remove the remaining shaving cream. ☑☐

13. Dry the person's face with the towel that is covering his chest. ☑☐

14. Give the person a hand mirror so that he can inspect the shaved area. ☑☐

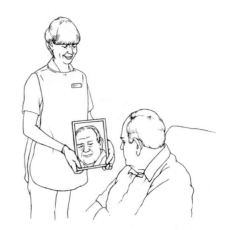

15. Assist the person to apply after-shave lotion, if he prefers it. ☑☐

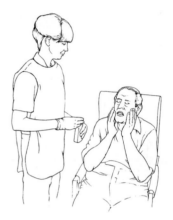

Why? Alcohol in after-shave helps to keep germs from growing because it acts as an antiseptic on any tiny cuts and scrapes, or abrasions. Also, when after-shave dries, or evaporates, it causes a cooling sensation that some people find refreshing.

Note: Put the razor in the sharps container or, if it is reusable, place it blade end down in a container. Do not recap.

16. Take off the gloves and throw them away. ☐☐

17. Raise the side rail, if used. ☑☐

Completion

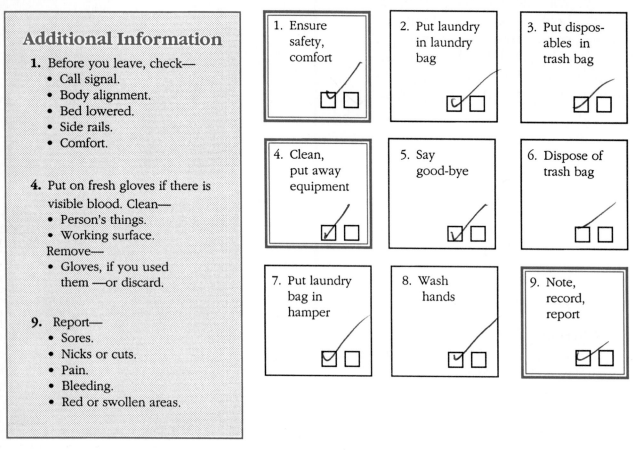

1. Ensure safety, comfort

2. Put laundry in laundry bag

3. Put disposables in trash bag

4. Clean, put away equipment

5. Say good-bye

6. Dispose of trash bag

7. Put laundry bag in hamper

8. Wash hands

9. Note, record, report

Student

Instructor

Date

Date

Martha Gromeka 7/11/94

130

Skill 29: Helping a Man Shave with an Electric Razor

Precautions

- Use electric razors instead of safety razors on all people with blood-clotting disorders or on people undergoing special drugs that change how fast the blood clots.
- Always ask the supervising nurse if a person should be shaved.
- Check to see if razor is in good shape; the screen has no holes, the cord is not frayed.
- Use an electric razor only in a room where no one is receiving oxygen. If oxygen is present, you could set off a spark and start a fire.

Preparation

1. Gather supplies
   - Towel
   - Washcloth
   - Laundry bag (or plastic bag for wet or soiled linens)

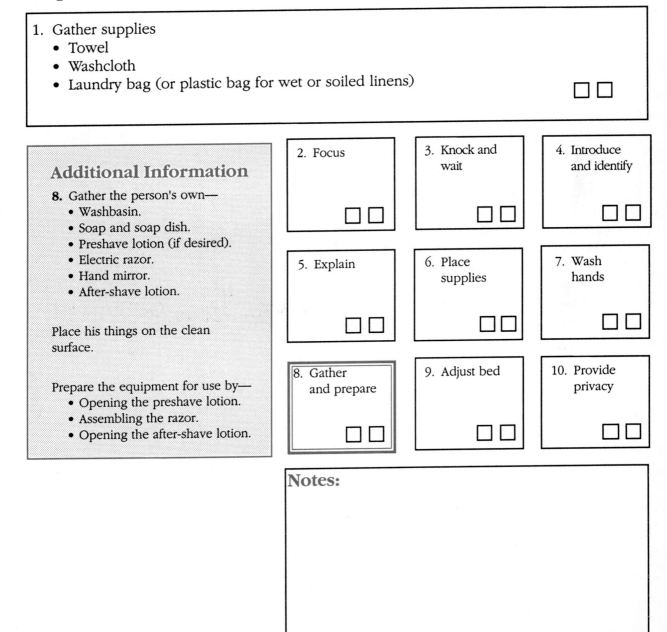

Additional Information

8. Gather the person's own—
- Washbasin.
- Soap and soap dish.
- Preshave lotion (if desired).
- Electric razor.
- Hand mirror.
- After-shave lotion.

Place his things on the clean surface.

Prepare the equipment for use by—
- Opening the preshave lotion.
- Assembling the razor.
- Opening the after-shave lotion.

2. Focus

3. Knock and wait

4. Introduce and identify

5. Explain

6. Place supplies

7. Wash hands

8. Gather and prepare

9. Adjust bed

10. Provide privacy

Notes:

Procedure

1. Fill the washbasin with warm water. Use a paper towel to turn the faucet on and off. Place the basin on the clean surface. Check the temperature of the water to see if it is warm to the touch on the inside of your wrist. ☐ ☐

2. Lower the side rail, if used, on the side of the bed where you are working. ☐ ☐

3. Help the person into a sitting position. ☐ ☐

Note: If the person is unconscious, elevate his head slightly.

4. Place the towel over his chest. ☐ ☐

5. Inspect the person's skin for moles, birthmarks, or sores. ☐ ☐

6. Using the washbasin of warm water, allow the person to wash his face, if he is able. Use soap, if he prefers, and remove the soap, if used, with the wet washcloth. ☐ ☐

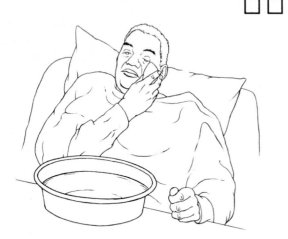

7. Help the person put pre-shave lotion on his face. ☐ ☐

Why? Pre-shave lotion softens the beard and helps the razor glide over the skin.

8. With the fingers of one hand, hold the person's skin tight as you use the razor to shave as the manufacturer suggests—usually in a circular motion. ☐ ☐

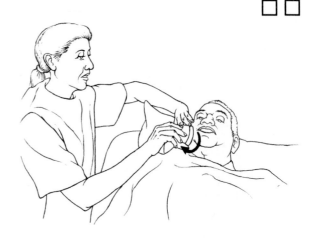

9. Work downward toward the person's neck under his chin. ☐ ☐

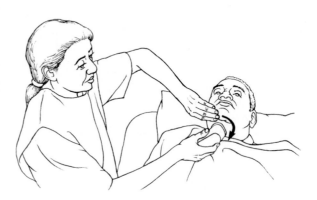

132

10. Use the wet washcloth to rinse the person's face. ☐ ☐

11. Dry the person's face with the towel that is covering his chest. ☐ ☐

12. Give the person a hand mirror so that he can inspect the shaved area. ☐ ☐

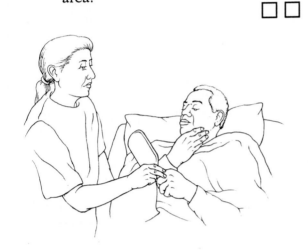

13. Apply after-shave lotion, if the person prefers it. ☐ ☐

14. Raise the side rail, if used. ☐ ☐

Completion

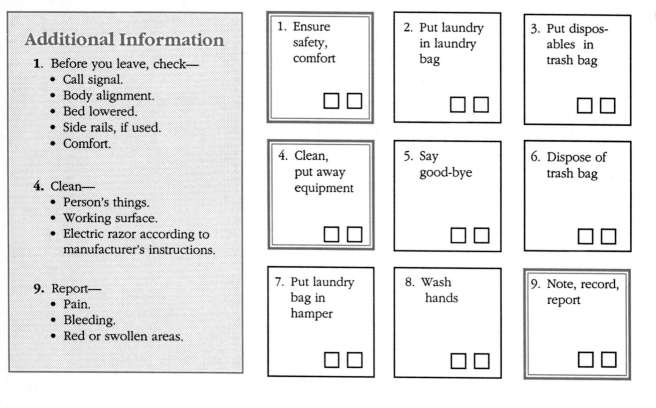

1. Ensure safety, comfort ☐ ☐

2. Put laundry in laundry bag ☐ ☐

3. Put disposables in trash bag ☐ ☐

4. Clean, put away equipment ☐ ☐

5. Say good-bye ☐ ☐

6. Dispose of trash bag ☐ ☐

7. Put laundry bag in hamper ☐ ☐

8. Wash hands ☐ ☐

9. Note, record, report ☐ ☐

_____
Student   Date

_____
Instructor   Date

Skill 30: Cleaning and Trimming a Person's Fingernails

Precautions

- Keep a person's fingernails trimmed and smooth to prevent injury to his skin.
- When trimming a person's fingernails, make sure his nails extend slightly beyond the tip of his fingers so that you do not injure the skin on his fingers.
- Use extra caution when you cut the fingernails of persons who have diabetes, poor circulation, paralysis (on paralyzed side), or decreased sensation in the hands.

Preparation

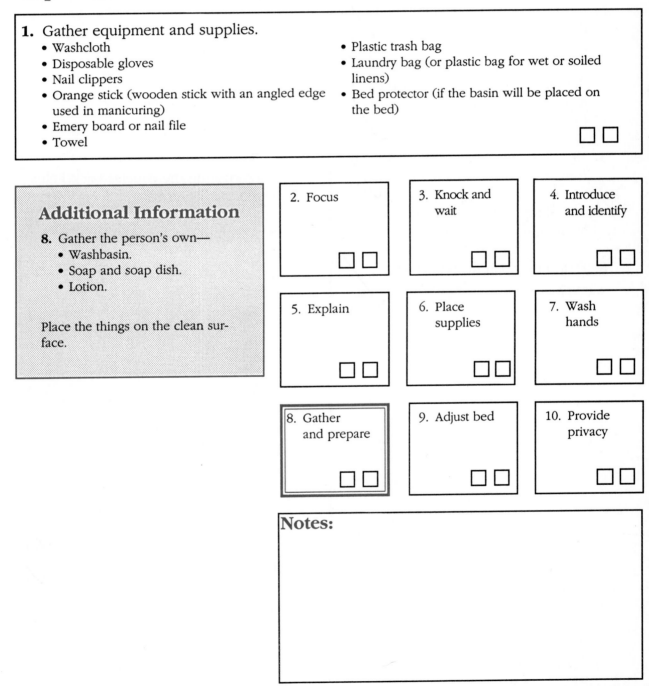

1. Gather equipment and supplies.
- Washcloth
- Disposable gloves
- Nail clippers
- Orange stick (wooden stick with an angled edge used in manicuring)
- Emery board or nail file
- Towel
- Plastic trash bag
- Laundry bag (or plastic bag for wet or soiled linens)
- Bed protector (if the basin will be placed on the bed)

☐ ☐

Additional Information

8. Gather the person's own—
- Washbasin.
- Soap and soap dish.
- Lotion.

Place the things on the clean surface.

2. Focus ☐ ☐

3. Knock and wait ☐ ☐

4. Introduce and identify ☐ ☐

5. Explain ☐ ☐

6. Place supplies ☐ ☐

7. Wash hands ☐ ☐

8. Gather and prepare ☐ ☐

9. Adjust bed ☐ ☐

10. Provide privacy ☐ ☐

Notes:

Procedure

1. Fill the washbasin with warm water and place it on a clean surface. Check the temperature of the water. ☑ ☐

2. Lower the side rail, if used, on the side of the bed where you are working. ☑ ☐

3. Help the person to a sitting position, if possible. ☐ ☐

4. Place the basin of water within the person's reach. Use bed protector if basin is placed on the bed. ☑ ☐

5. Help the person soak his hands in warm water for 5 minutes. ☑ ☐

Why? Soaking softens the nails and makes them easier to trim.

6. Help him wash his hands with soap. ☑ ☐

7. Lift his hands from the water, one at a time, and hold them over the washbasin as you push the skin at the base of the nails, or cuticles, back gently with a washcloth. ☑ ☐

Why? Pushing the cuticles back helps prevent hangnails.

8. Clean under the fingernails with the orange stick. ☑ ☐

9. Unfold a towel and rest the person's wet hands on it. ☑ ☐

10. Raise the side rail, if used. ☑ ☐

11. Empty the water from the wash-basin into the sink and wash the washbasin. Refill the washbasin with warm water and check the temperature of the water. ☑☐

12. Return with the fresh basin of water to the bed and lower the side rail, if used. ☑☐

13. Rinse the person's hands. ☑☐

Why? Rinsing the hands in clear, warm water won't dry and irritate the skin, as soapy water will.

14. Use the towel the person's hands were resting on to dry the person's hands thoroughly. Make sure the skin is dry between his fingers. ☐☐

Why? Drying the hands thoroughly helps prevent chapping.

15. Put on disposable gloves. Use nail clippers to cut the person's fingernails. Cut them straight across. ☑☐

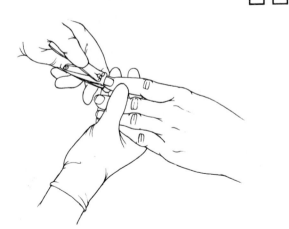

16. Remove the gloves and put them in the plastic trash bag. Use a nail file or an emery board to shape, trim, and smooth his fingernails, making sure there are no sharp edges when you finish. ☑☐

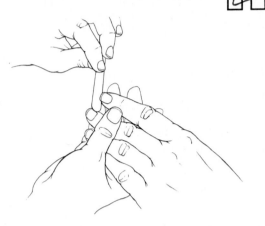

17. Put lotion on the person's hands. Gently massage his hands from the fingertips toward his wrist. ☑☐

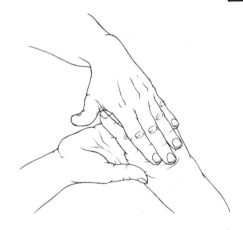

Why? Working in this direction helps to improve blood circulation. ☑☐

18. Raise the side rail, if used.

Completion

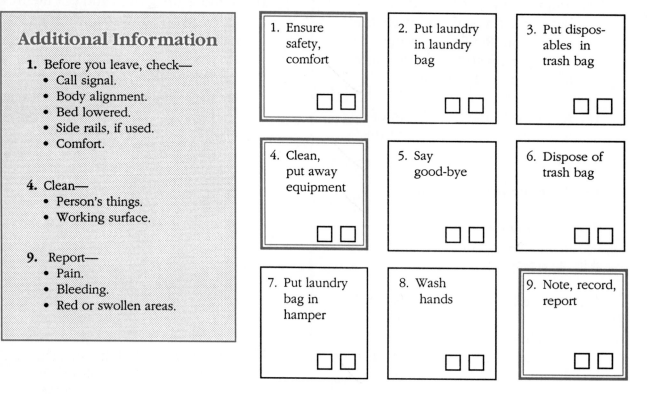

1. Ensure safety, comfort ☐ ☐

2. Put laundry in laundry bag ☐ ☐

3. Put disposables in trash bag ☐ ☐

4. Clean, put away equipment ☐ ☐

5. Say good-bye ☐ ☐

6. Dispose of trash bag ☐ ☐

7. Put laundry bag in hamper ☐ ☐

8. Wash hands ☐ ☐

9. Note, record, report ☐ ☐

_____

Student   Date

_____

Instructor   Date

Skill 31: Providing Foot Care and Cleaning a Person's Toenails

Precautions

- Although you provide a person with general foot and toenail care, only a doctor or a nurse should cut a person's toenails because of the chance of injury from cutting nails too short or cutting the skin around the nail.

Preparation

1. Gather supplies
   - Disposable bed protector
   - Towel
   - Washcloth
   - Plastic trash bag
   - Laundry bag (or plastic bag for wet or soiled linens) ☐ ☐

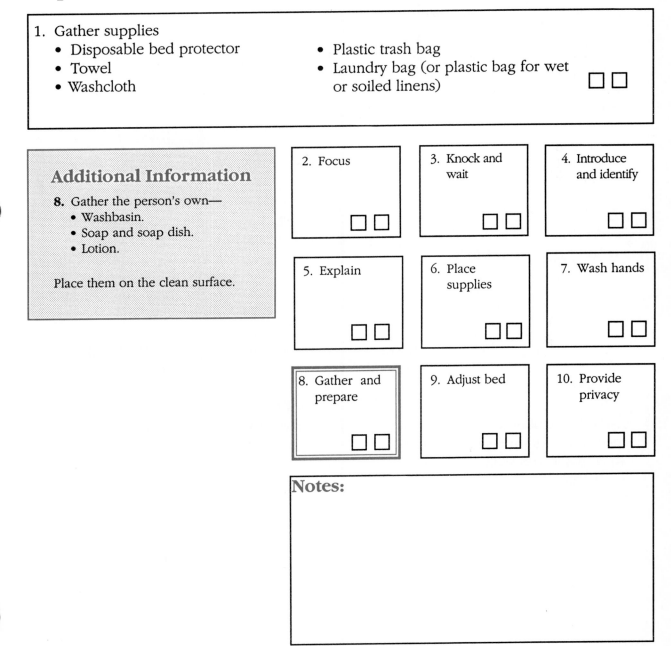

Additional Information

8. Gather the person's own—
   - Washbasin.
   - Soap and soap dish.
   - Lotion.

Place them on the clean surface.

2. Focus ☐ ☐

3. Knock and wait ☐ ☐

4. Introduce and identify ☐ ☐

5. Explain ☐ ☐

6. Place supplies ☐ ☐

7. Wash hands ☐ ☐

8. Gather and prepare ☐ ☐

9. Adjust bed ☐ ☐

10. Provide privacy ☐ ☐

Notes:

Procedure

1. Fill the washbasin with warm water and place it on a clean surface. Check the temperature of the water. ☐☐

2. Help the person out of bed and into a chair, if possible. ☐☐

Why? This position allows you to place the feet directly into the washbasin of water.

Note: If the person cannot get out of bed, help him lie flat or in a semi-Fowler's position. Place the washbasin on a bed protector near the person's foot. Flex the person's knee and place his foot into the basin.

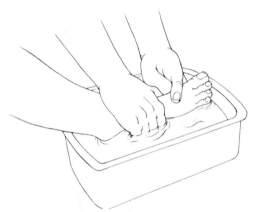

3. Place a disposable bed protector on the floor in front of the person. ☐☐

Note: Remember to use proper body mechanics. Sit on a short stool or squat while you work on the person's feet.

4. Place the washbasin on the bed protector. ☐☐

5. Help the person soak his feet for at least 5 minutes. ☐☐

Why? Soaking loosens dirt under the nails and make them easier to clean.

6. Help the person wash his feet with a soapy washcloth. ☐☐

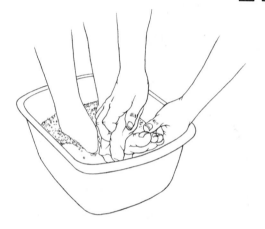
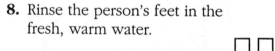

7. Empty the washbasin into the sink and rinse it out. Refill it with warm water and check the temperature to see that it is warm to the touch on the inside of your wrist. ☐☐

8. Rinse the person's feet in the fresh, warm water. ☐☐

Why? Rinsing the feet in clear, warm water won't dry and irritate the skin, as soapy water will.

9. Unfold a towel. Use it to dry the person's feet thoroughly, especially between the toes. Use the towel to gently push back the person's cuticles as you dry his foot. □ □

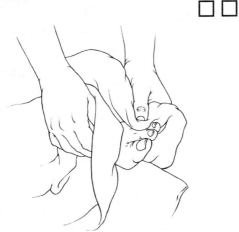

Why? Any moisture between toes can cause skin breakdown.

10. Inspect the condition of the skin on the person's feet, including between all toes. □ □

11. Put lotion on your hands. Gently massage the person's feet with the lotion. Begin with his toes and move upward toward his leg, but massage only his feet, not his legs. □ □

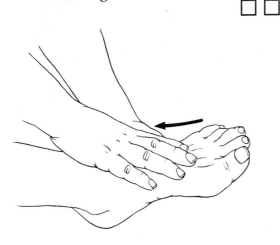

Why? Working in this direction, from the toes to the legs, helps to improve blood circulation. Massaging the calves of his legs could dangerously dislodge blood clots if any are present.

12. Help the person put on clean socks and shoes. □ □

13. If the person is staying in bed, raise the side rail, if used. □ □

Completion

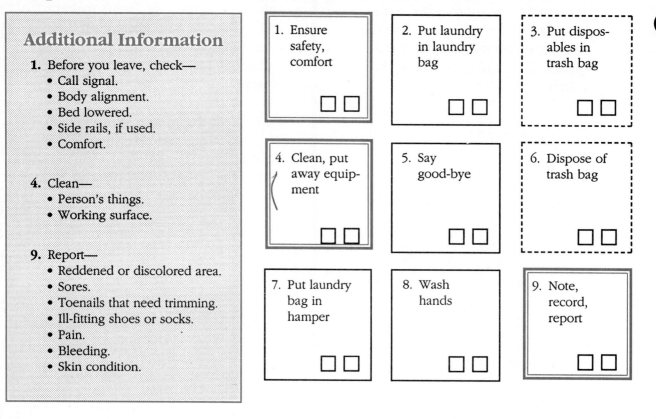

Additional Information

1. Before you leave, check—
   - Call signal.
   - Body alignment.
   - Bed lowered.
   - Side rails, if used.
   - Comfort.

4. Clean—
   - Person's things.
   - Working surface.

9. Report—
   - Reddened or discolored area.
   - Sores.
   - Toenails that need trimming.
   - Ill-fitting shoes or socks.
   - Pain.
   - Bleeding.
   - Skin condition.

1. Ensure safety, comfort ☐ ☐

2. Put laundry in laundry bag ☐ ☐

3. Put disposables in trash bag ☐ ☐

4. Clean, put away equipment ☐ ☐

5. Say good-bye ☐ ☐

6. Dispose of trash bag ☐ ☐

7. Put laundry bag in hamper ☐ ☐

8. Wash hands ☐ ☐

9. Note, record, report ☐ ☐

_____
Student   Date

Martha Grossv   7/1/G4
Instructor   Date

Skill 32: Helping a Person Undress

Precautions

- To avoid the possibility of the person's falling, make sure he sits down when taking off his clothing.
- To provide privacy and warmth, keep the person covered as much as possible while he undresses.

Preparation

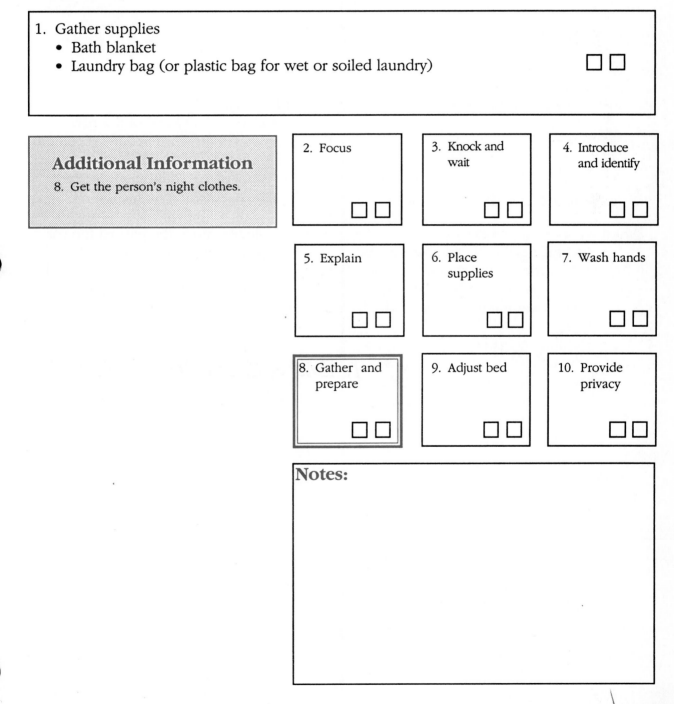

1. Gather supplies
   - Bath blanket
   - Laundry bag (or plastic bag for wet or soiled laundry)   ☐ ☐

Additional Information

8. Get the person's night clothes.

2. Focus   ☐ ☐

3. Knock and wait   ☐ ☐

4. Introduce and identify   ☐ ☐

5. Explain   ☐ ☐

6. Place supplies   ☐ ☐

7. Wash hands   ☐ ☐

8. Gather and prepare   ☐ ☐

9. Adjust bed   ☐ ☐

10. Provide privacy   ☐ ☐

Notes:

Procedure

1. Help the person sit on the side of the bed. ☐ ☐

2. Help him take off his shirt (or her dress). If the person has a weak or paralyzed side, remove the clothing from the strong or unaffected side first. ☐ ☐

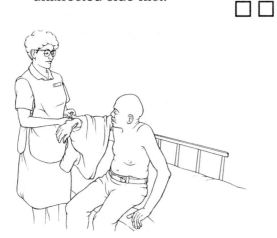

If the person has an IV:
- Carefully gather the clothing material, starting at the shoulder of the sleeve that has the IV. Glide the sleeve over the needle site and tubing.
- Holding the gathered sleeve, carefully unhook the IV bottle from the IV pole and slide the tubing, the bag, and your hand through the gathered sleeve. Hook the IV bottle back on the IV pole.

Note: Be very careful of the IV insertion site.

3. Cover him, as necessary, with the bath blanket. ☐ ☐

4. Help him take off his undershirt (or her bra and slip). ☐ ☐

5. Help him put on his pajama top (or her nightgown). ☐ ☐ ●

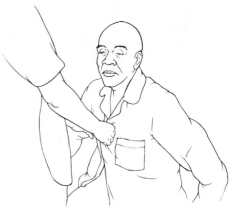

If he has an IV:
- Gather the sleeve of the pajama top (or gown) that will be going on the arm with the IV. Carefully unhook the IV bottle from the pole. Slide the bottle, the tubing, and the person's arm through the sleeve. Move the pajama top (or gown) up to the person's shoulder. ☐ ☐ ●

6. Help him take off his shoes and socks. ☐ ☐

7. Help him lie down in bed, and cover him with the bath blanket.

8. Help him remove his underpants and pants. Ask him to raise his hips so that you can reach under the bath blanket to help slip the pants down over his hips. ☐ ☐

●

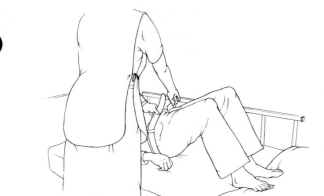

For clarity, the bath blanket has been omitted from the drawings.

Note: If a person can't raise his hips to wiggle out of his underpants and pants while lying down in a supine position—

- Unfasten the zipper, buttons, or ties as needed.
- Turn the person on his side and pull his pants over his buttocks and hip on that side.
- Repeat the process on his other side by turning him onto his other hip.
- Turn the person back into a supine position.

9. Help the person put on his pajama bottoms. Ask him to raise his hips so that you can reach under the bath blanket to help slip the bottoms up over his hips. Remove the bath blanket. ☐ ☐

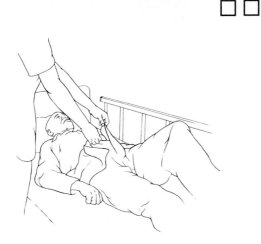

Note: If a person can't raise his hips to wiggle into his pajama bottoms while lying down in a supine position—

- Turn the person on his side and pull his pajama bottoms over his buttocks and hip on that side.
- Repeat process on his other side by turning him onto his other hip.
- Turn the person back into a supine position.

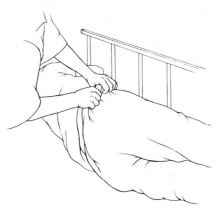

10. Make sure the person's night clothes are smooth and not bunched up.

   ☐ ☐

11. Raise the side rails, if used.

   ☐ ☐

Completion

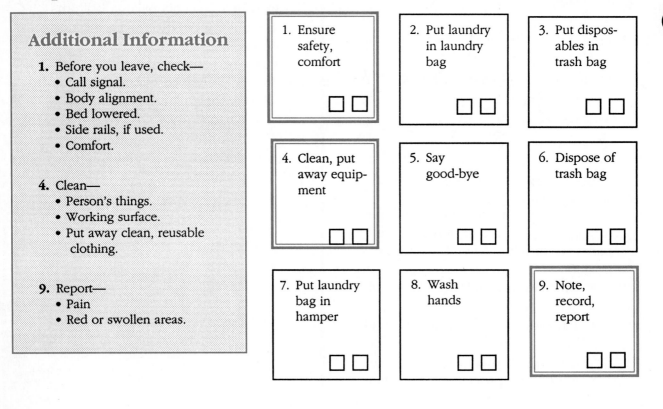

Additional Information

1. Before you leave, check—
- Call signal.
- Body alignment.
- Bed lowered.
- Side rails, if used.
- Comfort.

4. Clean—
- Person's things.
- Working surface.
- Put away clean, reusable clothing.

9. Report—
- Pain
- Red or swollen areas.

1. Ensure safety, comfort ☐ ☐

2. Put laundry in laundry bag ☐ ☐

3. Put disposables in trash bag ☐ ☐

4. Clean, put away equipment ☐ ☐

5. Say good-bye ☐ ☐

6. Dispose of trash bag ☐ ☐

7. Put laundry bag in hamper ☐ ☐

8. Wash hands ☐ ☐

9. Note, record, report ☐ ☐

_____

Student   Date

_____

Instructor   Date

Skill 33: Helping a Person Dress

Precautions

- To avoid the possibility of the person's falling, make sure he sits down when putting on his clothing.
- Make sure the person is dressed appropriately for the weather and situation.
- To provide privacy and warmth, keep the person covered as much as possible while he dresses.

Preparation

1. Gather supplies
   - Bath blanket
   - Laundry bag (or plastic bag for wet of soiled laundry) ☐ ☐

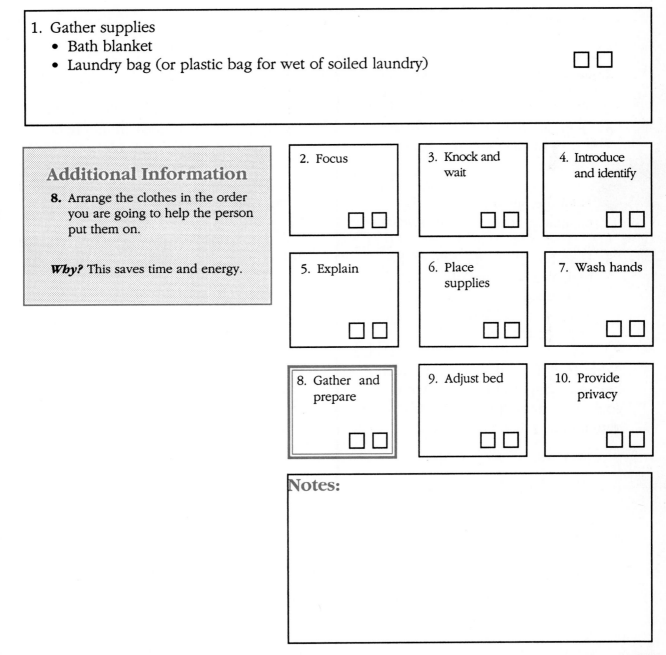

Additional Information

8. Arrange the clothes in the order you are going to help the person put them on.

Why? This saves time and energy.

2. Focus ☐ ☐	3. Knock and wait ☐ ☐	4. Introduce and identify ☐ ☐
5. Explain ☐ ☐	6. Place supplies ☐ ☐	7. Wash hands ☐ ☐
8. Gather and prepare ☐ ☐	9. Adjust bed ☐ ☐	10. Provide privacy ☐ ☐

Notes:

Procedure

1. Encourage him to choose the clothes he wears. ☐ ☐

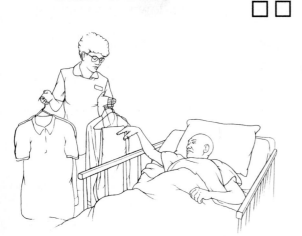

2. Lower the side rail, if used, on the side where you are working. ☐ ☐

3. Help him lie flat. Cover him with a bath blanket and pull back the top sheet. ☐ ☐

4. Help the person remove his pajama bottoms (or underwear). ☐ ☐

5. Help him sit on the side of the bed, and help him put on socks (or her stockings). Keep the lower part of his body covered with the bath blanket. ☐ ☐

Note: Look for red spots on his feet before putting on his socks. Avoid socks with tight upper elastic (or garters) that impair circulation.

6. Help him put on underwear and pants part way. To do this, have the person put both legs in the legs of both the underpants and the pants while sitting. ☐ ☐

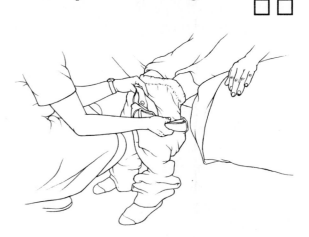

7. Help him put on his shoes. Make sure that his shoes are not tight and do not squeeze his toes. Help him stand. ☐ ☐

8. Help the person pull up his underwear and pants. ☐ ☐

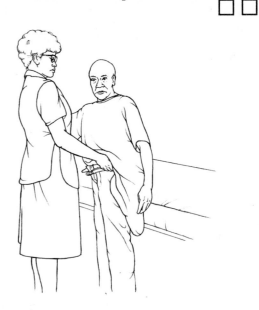

9. Help the person sit back down. ☐ ☐

Why? It's easier to finish dressing while the person is sitting down.

Note: If a person can't sit up for dressing, help him lie in a supine position and—

- Put both legs into the legs of the underpants and pants.
- Turn him on his side and pull his pants over his buttocks and hip on that side.
- Repeat the process on other side by turning him onto his other hip.
- Turn him back into a supine position.
- Fasten the zipper, buttons, or ties as needed.

10. If the person is female, adjust the bath blanket so that it covers her shoulders and upper body. Remove her gown from underneath the bath blanket to avoid exposing her. If the gown must come off over her head, pull it off one arm at a time while she uses the other arm to hold the bath blanket over herself. Help her hook her bra in front and turn it around so the hooks are in the back. ☐ ☐

Why? It is easier to see the hooks when they are in the front.

See Skill 32 for instructions on helping a person with an IV undress.

Reach under the bath blanket, as necessary, to help the person put her arms through the bra shoulder straps. Remove the bath blanket.

11. Help the person put his arms into the armholes of his undershirt (or her slip). Smooth out his undershirt (or her slip) across the back. ☐ ☐

Note: If the person has a weak or paralyzed arm, put that arm in the sleeve first.

Note: If the person has an IV, make sure that the sleeves of the clothing are large enough for the IV bag or bottle. See Skill 32 for instructions on helping a person with an IV.

12. Help him put his arms into the sleeves of his shirt (or her dress). Smooth out the back of his shirt (or her dress) and fasten it. ☐ ☐

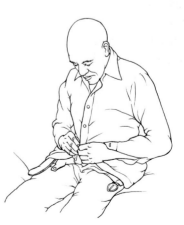

Note: Allow the person to do as much as possible for himself.

13. Help him stand again so that you can help tuck in the shirt and fasten or zip the pants. ☐ ☐

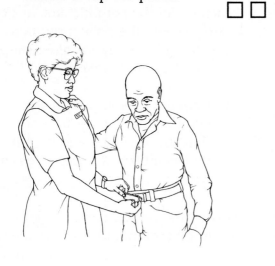

14. Help the person with accessories, such as a belt, scarf, or jewelry, if he or she asks you. ☐ ☐

15. If he wants to remain in bed, raise the side rail, if used. ☐ ☐

Completion

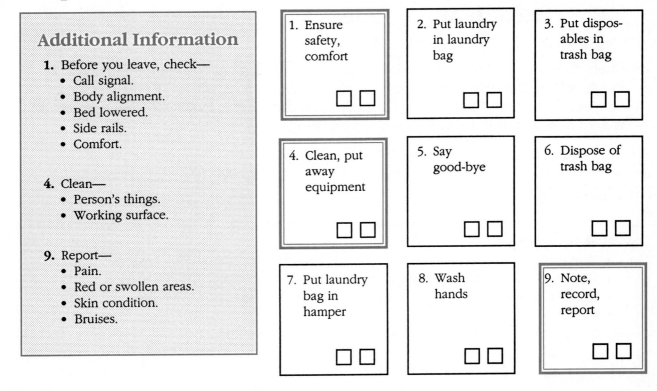

Additional Information

1. Before you leave, check—
   - Call signal.
   - Body alignment.
   - Bed lowered.
   - Side rails.
   - Comfort.

4. Clean—
   - Person's things.
   - Working surface.

9. Report—
   - Pain.
   - Red or swollen areas.
   - Skin condition.
   - Bruises.

1. Ensure safety, comfort ☐ ☐

2. Put laundry in laundry bag ☐ ☐

3. Put disposables in trash bag ☐ ☐

4. Clean, put away equipment ☐ ☐

5. Say good-bye ☐ ☐

6. Dispose of trash bag ☐ ☐

7. Put laundry bag in hamper ☐ ☐

8. Wash hands ☐ ☐

9. Note, record, report ☐ ☐

_____

Student   Date

_____

Instructor   Date

Skill 34: Assisting with Medications—The Home Health Aide's Role

Precautions

- Check the prescription label. Make sure you have the right client, the right medication, the right time, the right amount, and the right route.
- Let your supervising nurse know if a medication container is missing a label or if the label is hard to read and if the medication has expired.

Preparation

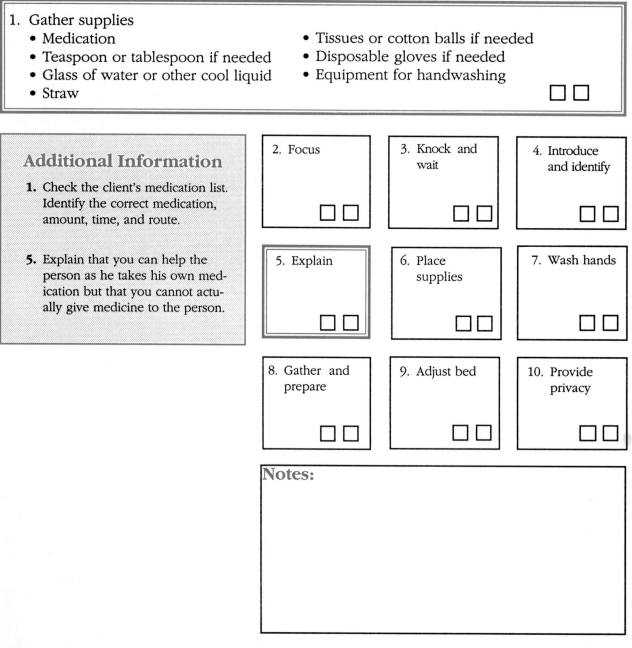

1. Gather supplies
   - Medication
   - Teaspoon or tablespoon if needed
   - Glass of water or other cool liquid
   - Straw
   - Tissues or cotton balls if needed
   - Disposable gloves if needed
   - Equipment for handwashing
   ☐ ☐

Additional Information

1. Check the client's medication list. Identify the correct medication, amount, time, and route.

5. Explain that you can help the person as he takes his own medication but that you cannot actually give medicine to the person.

2. Focus ☐ ☐

3. Knock and wait ☐ ☐

4. Introduce and identify ☐ ☐

5. Explain ☐ ☐

6. Place supplies ☐ ☐

7. Wash hands ☐ ☐

8. Gather and prepare ☐ ☐

9. Adjust bed ☐ ☐

10. Provide privacy ☐ ☐

Notes:

Procedure

1. Provide privacy for the person. Ask visitors to leave the room. ☐ ☐

2. Help the client wash his hands. ☐ ☐

3. Place the medications within the client's reach. Make sure the client has his eyeglasses, if they are needed. ☐ ☐

4. Loosen container lids, tops, or caps. Tell the client the names of each medication. ☐ ☐

5. Assist the client with oral medications (tablets, capsules, liquids) as necessary:

   • Support the client's hand if necessary as he pours medication into a spoon, cup, or other hand.
   • Give the client the glass of water.

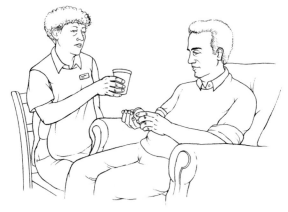

   • Make sure the client swallows the medication. ☐ ☐

6. Help the client with eye medications as necessary:
   • Position the client so that her head is tilted back.

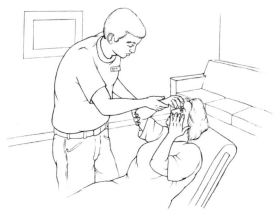

   • Know which eye will receive the medication.
   • Support the client's hand as she drops the medication into the lower eyelid.
   • Ask the client to close her eyes to help distribute the medication. ☐ ☐

7. Assist the client with topical medications (ointments, lotions) as necessary:
   • Help him remove any dressing.
   • Wash the area as instructed by your supervisor.
   • Have the client apply the medication.

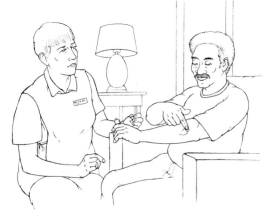

   • Help him with handwashing. ☐ ☐

153

8. Help the client with a rectal suppository as necessary:

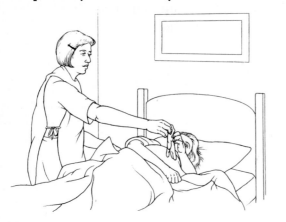

- Help the client to a side-lying position.
- Help the client unwrap the suppository.
- Ask the client to put on a disposable glove.
- Guide the client's hand to the rectal area, if necessary.
- Have the client insert the suppository.
- Hold his buttocks together for a few minutes.

Why? This will help the client retain the suppository.

- Help the client assume a comfortable position.

☐ ☐

Completion

Additional Information

1. Before you leave, check—
- Call signal.
- Body alignment.
- Bed lowered.
- Side rails, if used.
- Comfort.

9. Report—
- The medication taken, the amount, the time, and the route.
- Any difficulties the client had in taking the medication (difficulty swallowing, hand tremors).
- Any observed side effects or client complaints.

Notify your supervising nurse if your client—
- Is not taking his medication as prescribed.
- Is taking more or less than the prescribed amount.
- Is taking drugs other than those prescribed, including over-the-counter drugs.
- Is mixing up prescribed medications.
- Is taking his medication at times other than those ordered.
- Has any questions concerning his medications.

Also let your supervising nurse know—
- When your client has 1 week of pills left from a prescription.

Why? The strength of expired medications cannot be guaranteed.
- If you suspect that anyone in the household is misusing drugs.

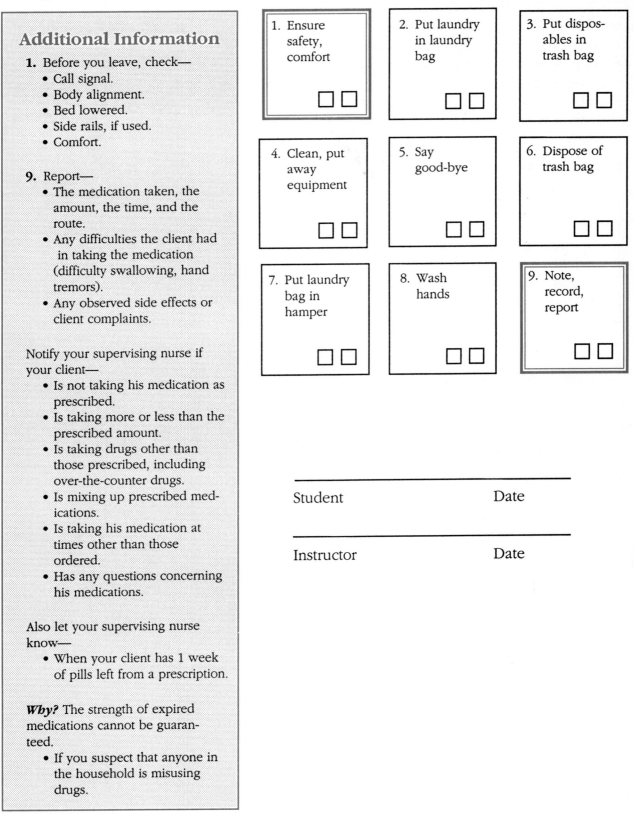

1. Ensure safety, comfort

2. Put laundry in laundry bag

3. Put disposables in trash bag

4. Clean, put away equipment

5. Say good-bye

6. Dispose of trash bag

7. Put laundry bag in hamper

8. Wash hands

9. Note, record, report

Student   Date

Instructor   Date

Skill 35: Making an Unoccupied Bed

Precautions

- Keep clean linens on a clean surface.
- Keep clean and dirty linens from touching the floor.
- Remove and replace linens carefully, without shaking them. Shaking linens causes air currents that may spread dust and germs around the room.
- Keep dirty, contaminated linens away from your uniform.
- Use proper body mechanics.

Preparation

1. Gather supplies
   To save time and energy, stack linens in this order so that the item you use last is on the bottom of the pile.
   - Pillowcase
   - Top sheet
   - Drawsheet
   - Bottom sheet
   - Laundry bag (or plastic bag for wet or soiled linens) ☐ ☐

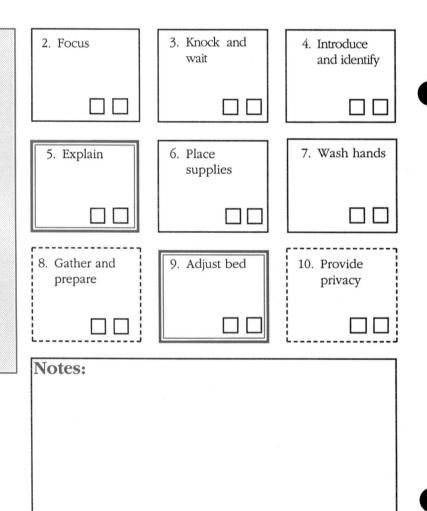

Additional Information

1. Wash your hands before gathering clean linens.
- Take only the linens you need into the person's room. In a hospital or nursing home, any linens you take into a person's room have to be laundered. They cannot be used for another person.

5. Ask the person to sit in a chair while you make the bed.

9. The bed should be flat and raised. Bend your knees if the bed cannot be raised.

2. Focus ☐ ☐

3. Knock and wait ☐ ☐

4. Introduce and identify ☐ ☐

5. Explain ☐ ☐

6. Place supplies ☐ ☐

7. Wash hands ☐ ☐

8. Gather and prepare ☐ ☐

9. Adjust bed ☐ ☐

10. Provide privacy ☐ ☐

Notes:

Procedure

The four tasks for making an unoccupied bed are:

1. Removing dirty linens
2. Placing clean and reusable linens on the first side of the bed
3. Placing clean and reusable linens on the second side of the bed
4. Placing clean linens on the pillow

Task 1: Removing Dirty Linens

1. Lower the side rails, if used. ☐ ☐

2. Check the dirty bed linens for personal items the person may have left in bed. (Some people may have items such as dentures, eyeglasses, or hearing aids in their beds.) ☐ ☐

   Why? Personal items may be costly or impossible to replace if they are lost or broken.

3. If you find any personal items in the bed, tell the person you need to move his personal things to a safe place where he can find them. Ask him where he would like you to put them. ☐ ☐

4. Loosen all sheets while moving around the bed. ☐ ☐

Why? Reaching across the bed instead of moving around it can strain your back, because you cannot keep your back straight while reaching.

5. Take the dirty pillowcase off the pillow and put it in the laundry bag. Place the pillow on a clean surface. ☐ ☐

Note: As you work, talk with the person. Encourage him to talk.

6. Take off reusable linens, such as the unsoiled blanket and spread. Fold the reusable linens and put them in a clean place, such as over the back of a clean chair. ☐ ☐

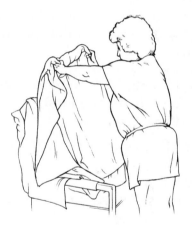

Why? Folding the reusable linens at this point to put back on the bed later saves time and energy.

7. Roll all dirty linens tightly and put them in the laundry bag. ☐ ☐

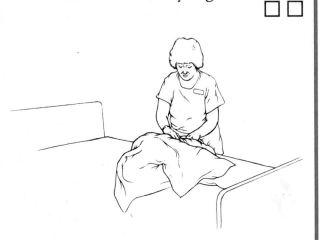

Why? Rolling the dirty linens tightly and putting them directly in the laundry bag help prevent the spread of germs.

Task 2: Placing Clean and Reusable Linens on the First Side of the Bed

1. Put the clean bottom sheet on the bed. ☐ ☐

For linens folded by a laundry:
With the center fold in the center of the bed and the narrow hem at the foot of the mattress along the edge, unfold the sheet away from you. Make sure the smooth side of the hem is on top, with the seam on the under side.

For linens laundered at home:
Fold the sheet in half lengthwise. Place the center fold in the center of the bed and the narrow hem at the foot of the mattress along the edge. Make sure the smooth side of the hem is on top, with the seam on the under side.

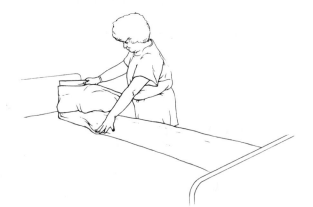

Why? This allows for enough fabric to be tucked in at the top and sides of the mattress. This also prevents the seam edge from irritating the person's skin.

Note: Open the sheets gently without shaking them. Shaking causes air currents that may spread dust and germs around the room.

Note: Some nursing homes, hospitals, and private homes use fitted bottom sheets instead of flat sheets.

2. Tuck in the sheet at the head of the mattress. ☐ ☐

3. Prepare a tight-fitting corner by mitering the corner, using the following steps:

- Face the head of the bed with your side next to the bed. With the hand that is next to the bed, lift the edge of the sheet at the side of the bed about 12 inches from the top of the mattress, making a triangle.

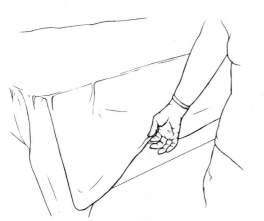

- Lay the triangle on top of the bed, holding the top of the triangle firmly.

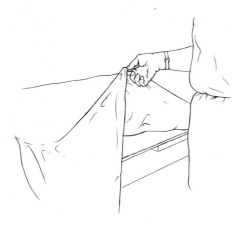

- Tuck the hanging portion of the sheet under the mattress.

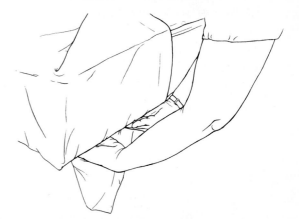

- Bring the triangle down and tuck it in. With your palms facing up, continue tucking in the sheet on the side, all the way to the foot of the mattress. ☐ ☐

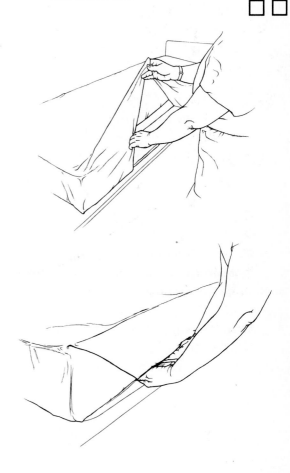

Why? A mitered corner makes the bed look neat. It also helps prevent the linens from becoming loose and wrinkled.

Why? When you keep your palms facing up while tucking in the sheets, you prevent yourself from injuring your wrist.

4. Place the drawsheet on the middle of the mattress with the center fold in the center of the bed. Unfold the drawsheet. With your palms facing up, tuck the drawsheet under the side of the mattress, tucking in the middle third first, then the top third, and then the bottom third. ☐ ☐

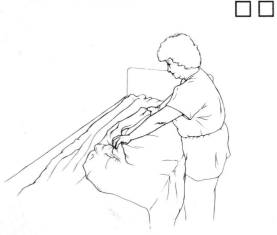

Why? By tucking the sections of the sheet in this order, the linens stay tucked in tightly.

Note: Be sure to move so that you stand in front of the section of the drawsheet you are tucking.

Why? Moving as you tuck prevents you from twisting your upper body.

For a home environment: Make a drawsheet by folding a flat sheet in half crosswise.

5. Put the clean top sheet on the bed with the center fold in the center. Place the wide hem even with the head of the mattress, with the seam on the outside. ☐ ☐

Why? By placing the center fold in the center, the sheet hangs evenly on both sides. Also, the bed looks neater. By placing the seam on the outside, the rough part of the hem won't touch the person's skin.

6. Remove the folded blanket from the back of the chair. Unfold it. Place the blanket over the top sheet about 6 inches down from the top edge. ☐ ☐

Why? This allows room for the sheet to be turned down over the blanket.

Place it with the center fold in the center so that the sides hang evenly.

7. Remove the folded spread from the back of the chair. Unfold it. Place the spread over the blanket. Place it with the center fold in the center so that the sides hang evenly. ☐ ☐

8. Tuck in the top sheet, blanket, and spread together under the foot of the mattress. Miter the corners together. Do not tuck in the sides as you did with the bottom sheet. □ □

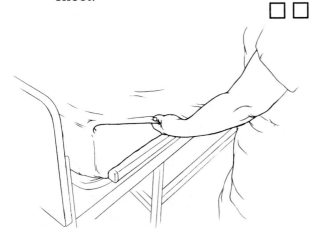

9. Fold the top of the spread down far enough so that there is room to cover the pillow. □ □

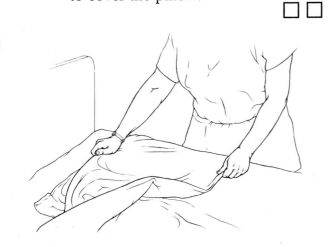

Task 3: Placing Clean and Reusable Linens on the Second Side of the Bed

1. Move to the opposite side of the bed. □ □

2. Tuck in the bottom sheet at the head of the mattress. □ □

3. Miter the corner of the sheet. □ □

4. With your palms facing up, continue tucking in the sheet all the way to the foot of the bed. □ □

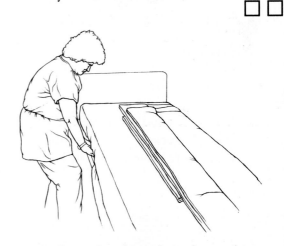

5. Tighten the drawsheet by tucking in the middle third first, then the top third, and then the bottom third. □ □

6. Straighten the top sheet. Tuck in the top sheet, blanket, and spread together under the foot of the mattress. Miter the corners together. Do not tuck in the sides, as you did with the bottom sheet. ☐ ☐

7. Fold the top of the spread down on each side of the bed far enough so that there is room to cover the pillow. ☐ ☐

8. Fold the top sheet down 6 inches over the blanket's edge on each side of the bed. ☐ ☐

Task 4: Placing Clean Linens on the Pillow

1. Hold the cover pillowcase at the center of the end seam. ☐ ☐

2. With your hand on the outside of the pillowcase, turn the pillowcase back over your hand. ☐ ☐

3. Hold the pillow through the pillowcase at the center of one end of the pillow. ☐ ☐

4. Bring the pillowcase down over the pillow. ☐ ☐

5. Fit the corners of the pillow into the corners of the pillowcase. ☐ ☐

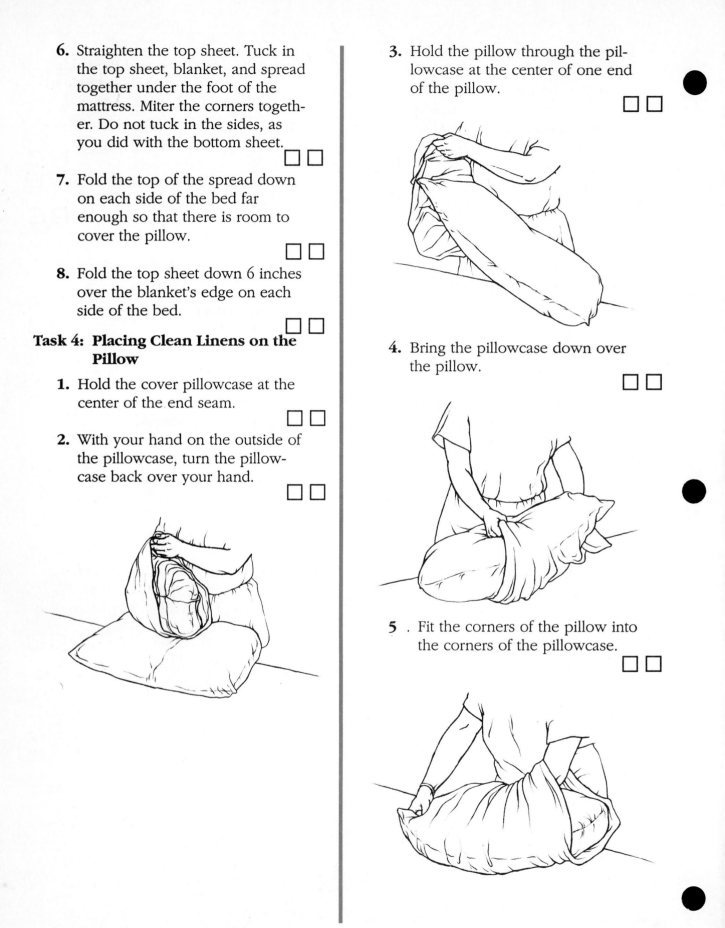

162

6. Put the pillow on the bed with the lower edge covering the fold of the bedspread. ☐ ☐

7. Cover the pillow with the bedspread (when the bed is completely made, this is called the closed position). ☐ ☐

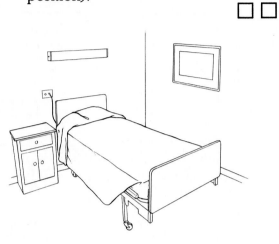

8. If the person is going back to bed, open the bed by fanfolding the linens to the foot of the bed and lowering the bed to its lowest position. Help the person into the bed and raise the side rail, if used. ☐ ☐

Completion

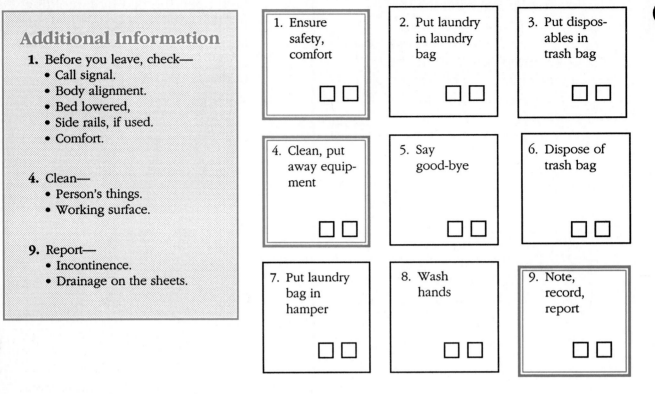

1. Ensure safety, comfort ☐ ☐

2. Put laundry in laundry bag ☐ ☐

3. Put disposables in trash bag ☐ ☐

4. Clean, put away equipment ☐ ☐

5. Say good-bye ☐ ☐

6. Dispose of trash bag ☐ ☐

7. Put laundry bag in hamper ☐ ☐

8. Wash hands ☐ ☐

9. Note, record, report ☐ ☐

_____

Student   Date

_____

Instructor   Date

Skill 36: Making an Occupied Bed

Precautions

- Keep the side rail up on the side where you are not working.
- Roll the person toward you, never away from you. There is less risk of injury to you and the person when you roll him toward you.
- Always stay with the person, never leaving him alone.
- Keep clean linens on a clean surface.
- Keep clean and dirty linens from touching the floor.
- Remove and replace linens carefully, without shaking them. Shaking linens causes air currents that may spread dust and germs around the room.
- Keep dirty, contaminated linens away from your uniform.

Preparation

1. Gather supplies
   To save time and energy, stack items in this order so that the item you use last is on the bottom of the pile:
   - Pillowcase
   - Top sheet
   - Drawsheet
   - Bottom sheet
   - Bath blanket (optional)
   - Extra sheet or bed protector (optional—use if you know the sheets are wet or soiled)
   - Laundry bag (or plastic bag for wet or soiled linens) ☐ ☐

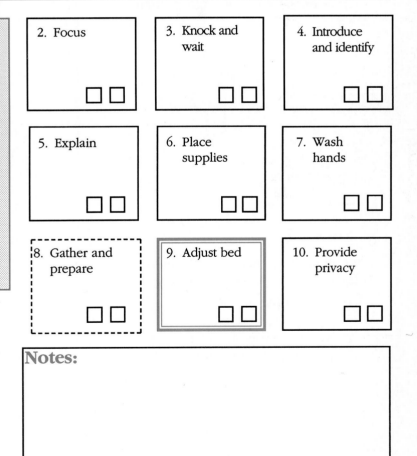

Additional Information

1. Wash your hands before gathering clean linens.
   - Take only the linens you need into the person's room.

9. The bed should be as flat as possible and raised. Some people may not be able to lie flat because it may make it hard for them to breathe. Bend your knees if the bed cannot be raised.

2. Focus ☐ ☐

3. Knock and wait ☐ ☐

4. Introduce and identify ☐ ☐

5. Explain ☐ ☐

6. Place supplies ☐ ☐

7. Wash hands ☐ ☐

8. Gather and prepare ☐ ☐

9. Adjust bed ☐ ☐

10. Provide privacy ☐ ☐

Notes:

Procedure

The five tasks for making an occupied bed are:

1. Removing and replacing linens on the first side of the bed.
2. Removing and replacing linens on the second side of the bed.
3. Removing and replacing linens on the pillow.
4. Replacing reusable linens.
5. Making a toe pleat.

Task 1: Removing and Replacing Linens on the First Side of the Bed

1. While moving around the bed, take off reusable linens, such as the unsoiled blanket and spread. Fold the reusable linens and put them in a clean place, such as over the back of a clean chair. ☐☐

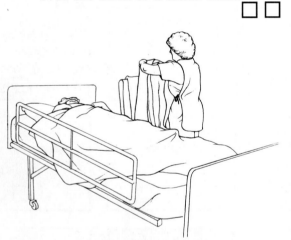

Why? Folding the reusable linens at this point to put back on the bed later saves time and energy.

2. Keep the top sheet on the person for privacy and warmth. ☐☐

Note: If the top sheet is wet or soiled, replace it with a bath blanket. Open up the bath blanket and place it over the person. Ask the person to hold onto the top edge while you remove the sheet from underneath. Place the wet or soiled sheet in the plastic bag.

3. Decide which side of the bed to make first. Make sure that the overbed table or nightstand, where you stacked the linens, is within reach. ☐☐

4. Go to the side of the bed that is opposite the side that you are going to make first. Before turning the person onto her side, check that side of the bed for personal items, such as dentures, eyeglasses, or hearing aids. If you find any, tell the person that you need to move her things to a safe place, and ask her where she would like you to put them. ☐☐

Why? Personal items may be costly or impossible to replace if they are lost or broken.

5. Lower the side rail, if used. Help the person roll toward you. Use the procedure you learned in Skill 13, Moving a Person Around in Bed, when turning the person toward you. Raise the side rail, if used. ☐☐

Note: The person can use the side rail for balance and support while you are making the bed.

6. Return to the opposite side of the bed, where you are working. Lower the side rail, if used. ☐ ☐

Note: To maintain the person's safety, lower the side rail only on the side where you are working. Also, if you must leave the bedside to put away something, remember to raise the side rail, if used.

7. Gently lift the person's head to adjust the pillow under her head to keep her comfortable. Check her for proper body alignment, signs of discomfort, and place-ment of drainage tubes. ☐ ☐

8. Check that side of the bed for personal items. If you find any, tell the person that you need to move her things to a safe place, and ask her where she would like you to put them. ☐ ☐

9. Loosen the dirty bottom sheet and draw sheet. Roll them toward the person and tuck them against her back. ☐ ☐

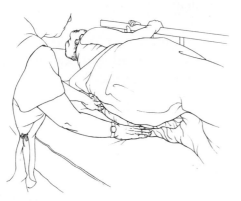

Note: If linens are soiled or there is any concern about infection control, put an extra sheet or bed protector around the soiled area to keep it away from the person and the clean sheets you are about to put on the bed.

10. Put the clean bottom sheet on the bed. ☐ ☐

For linens folded by a laundry:
With the center fold in the center of the bed and the narrow hem at the foot of the mattress along the edge, unfold the sheet away from you. Make sure the smooth side of the hem is on top, with the seam on the under side.

For linens laundered at home:
Fold the sheet in half lengthwise. Place the center fold in the center of the bed and the narrow hem at the foot of the mattress away from you. Unfold the sheet away from you. Make sure the smooth side of the hem is on top, with the seam on the under side.

Why? This allows for enough fabric to be tucked in at the top and sides of the mattress. This also prevents the seam edge from irritating the person's skin.

Note: Fanfold the top layer of the clean sheet next to the rolled dirty sheet.

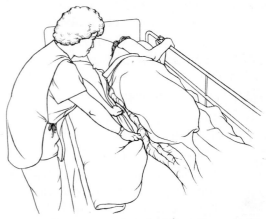

Note: Some nursing homes, hospitals, and private homes use fitted bottom sheets instead of flat sheets.

11. Tuck in the sheet at the head of the mattress. ☐ ☐

12. Prepare a tight-fitting corner by mitering the corner. ☐ ☐

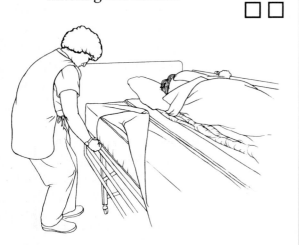

Note: Refer to mitering corners in Skill 35.

13. With your palms facing up, continue tucking in the sheet all the way to the foot of the mattress. ☐ ☐

14. Place the center fold of the drawsheet on the middle of the mattress. Fanfold the top layer of the drawsheet next to the rolled dirty sheet. With your palms facing up, tuck the remaining part under the side of the mattress, tucking in the middle third first, then the top third, and then the bottom third. ☐ ☐

15. Flatten the rolled dirty sheets as much as possible. Help the person roll over the dirty linens toward you. Adjust the pillow under the person's head. Check her for proper body alignment, signs of discomfort, and placement of drainage tubes. ☐ ☐

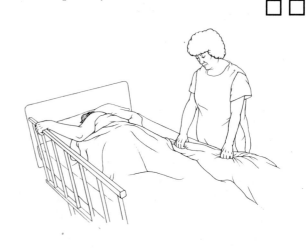

16. Raise the side rail, if used, on the side of the bed where you have been working. Then go to the opposite side of the bed. ☐ ☐

Task 2: Removing and Replacing Linens on the Second Side of the Bed

1. Lower the side rail, if used, on the side where you are working. ☐ ☐

2. Roll the dirty bottom sheets and put them in the laundry bag. ☐ ☐

Why? Use this technique so that the bed can be made completely without ever leaving the person.

3. Pull the clean, fanfolded bottom sheet toward you until it is completely unfolded. ☐ ☐

168

4. Tuck in the bottom sheet at the head of the mattress. ☐ ☐

5. Miter the corner of the sheet. ☐ ☐

6. With your palms facing up, continue tucking in the sheet all the way to the foot of the mattress. ☐ ☐

7. Pull the drawsheet out from under the person. Tighten it by tucking in the middle third first, then the top third, and then the bottom third. ☐ ☐

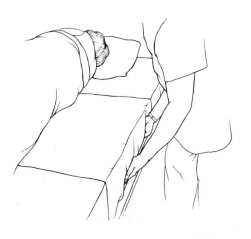

8. Help the person roll onto her back in the center of the bed. Adjust the pillow under her head. ☐ ☐

9. Put the clean top sheet over the dirty top sheet. Or, if you used a bath blanket to replace the wet top sheet, put the clean top sheet over the bath blanket. ☐ ☐

Why? You place the clean sheet over the person before removing the dirty sheet or the bath blanket to protect the person's privacy.

Place the wide hem of the sheet at the head with the smooth side of the hem next to the person. Be sure to put the center fold in the center so that the sides hang evenly and the top of the sheet is even with the top of the mattress.

10. Raise the side rail, if used. ☐ ☐

11. Have the person hold the clean top sheet in place while you remove the dirty sheet from underneath. Put the dirty sheet with the other dirty linens in the laundry bag or plastic bag. ☐ ☐

Task 3: Removing and Replacing Linens on the Pillow

1. Lower the side rail, if used, on the side where you are working. ☐ ☐

2. Carefully remove the pillow from under the person's head. ☐ ☐

3. Take the dirty pillowcase off the pillow and put it in the laundry bag. ☐ ☐

4. Hold the clean pillowcase at the center of the end seam. ☐ ☐

5. With your hand on the outside of the pillowcase, turn the pillowcase back over your hand. ☐ ☐

6. Hold the pillow through the pillowcase at the center of one end of the pillow. ☐ ☐

7. Bring the pillowcase down over the pillow. ☐ ☐

8. Fit the corners of the pillow into the corners of the pillowcase. ☐ ☐

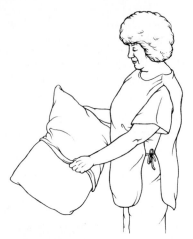

9. Gently lift the person's head to place the pillow under her head. ☐ ☐

10. Raise the side rail, if used. ☐ ☐

Task 4: Replacing Reusable Linens

1. Lower the side rail, if used, on the side where you will be working. Remove the folded blanket from the back of the chair. Work from one side of the bed to unfold and spread the blanket. Put the blanket over the top sheet about 6 inches down from the top of the mattress. Place it with the center fold in the center so that it hangs evenly. ☐ ☐

2. Remove the folded spread from the back of the chair. Work from one side of the bed to unfold and spread the bedspread. Place the spread over the blanket with the center fold in the center so that it hangs evenly, and the top hem even with the head of the mattress. ☐ ☐

3. Go to the foot of the bed to tuck in the top sheet, blanket, and spread together under the foot of the mattress. Miter the corners together. Do not tuck in the sides as you did with the bottom sheet. ☐ ☐

4. Fold the hem of the top sheet down over the blanket and spread. Fold the top sheet down 6 inches over the blanket and spread. Raise the side rail, if used. ☐ ☐

5. Complete the other side. ☐ ☐

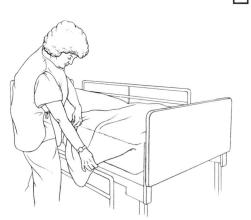

Task 5: Making a Toe Pleat

1. Standing at the foot of the bed, grasp both sides of the top covers about 18 inches from the foot of the bed. Gently pull the top covers toward the foot of the bed. ☐ ☐

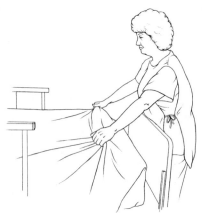

2. Make a 3- to 4-inch fold across the foot of the bed to make a toe pleat. ☐ ☐

Why? The toe pleat prevents pressure on the person's toes from the tight corners.

Completion

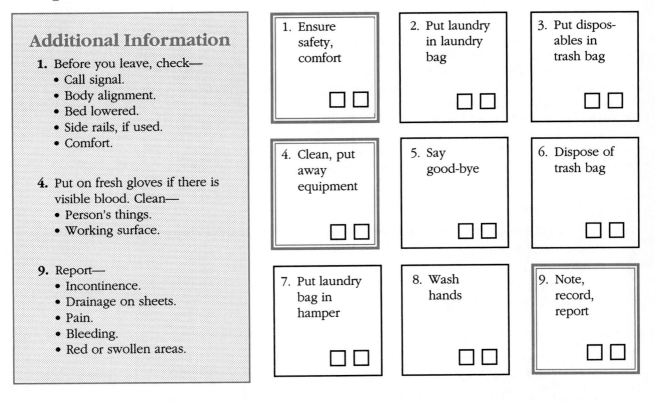

Additional Information

1. Before you leave, check—
- Call signal.
- Body alignment.
- Bed lowered.
- Side rails, if used.
- Comfort.

4. Put on fresh gloves if there is visible blood. Clean—
- Person's things.
- Working surface.

9. Report—
- Incontinence.
- Drainage on sheets.
- Pain.
- Bleeding.
- Red or swollen areas.

1. Ensure safety, comfort ☐ ☐

2. Put laundry in laundry bag ☐ ☐

3. Put disposables in trash bag ☐ ☐

4. Clean, put away equipment ☐ ☐

5. Say good-bye ☐ ☐

6. Dispose of trash bag ☐ ☐

7. Put laundry bag in hamper ☐ ☐

8. Wash hands ☐ ☐

9. Note, record, report ☐ ☐

Student _____ Date

Instructor _____ Date

Skill 37: Changing Crib Linens

Precautions

- Always stay with the infant, never leaving him alone.
- Keep clean linens on a clean surface.
- Keep clean and dirty linens from touching the floor.
- Remove and replace linens carefully, without shaking them. Shaking linens causes air currents that may spread dust and germs around the room.
- Keep dirty, contaminated linens away from your uniform.
- Use proper body mechanics.
- Be sure the top and bottom rails are in place if you must step away from the crib side.
- Keep one hand on the infant even if you are only turning away for a moment.
- Never use a pillow in an infant crib.

Preparation

1. Gather supplies
   - Bottom sheet
   - Baby blanket
   - Laundry bag (or plastic bag for wet or soiled linens) ☐ ☐

Additional Information

1. Wash your hands before gathering clean linens.

4. Talk to the infant as you work. Introduce yourself to the parent, if one is present.

5. Explain your tasks to the parent, if one is present.

---

2. Focus ☐ ☐

3. Knock and wait ☐ ☐

4. Introduce and identify ☐ ☐

5. Explain ☐ ☐

6. Place supplies ☐ ☐

7. Wash hands ☐ ☐

8. Gather and prepare ☐ ☐

9. Adjust bed ☐ ☐

10. Provide privacy ☐ ☐

Notes:

Procedure

1. Lower the side rail, if used, and raise the upper rail or cover if one is in place. ☐ ☐

2. Place the infant in a safe place, such as in a stroller or playpen, or ask the parent to hold the child. ☐ ☐

3. Remove the dirty sheet from the mattress and put it in the laundry bag. ☐ ☐

4. Place the clean sheet lengthwise on the side of the crib closer to you. ☐ ☐

5. Miter the top and bottom corners of the sheet (see Skill 35), or fit the corners of the fitted sheet around the mattress. ☐ ☐

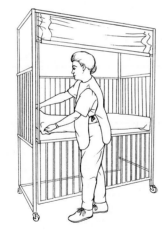

6. Raise the side rail, if used, and lower the upper rail or cover. Go around to the other side and lower the side rail and raise the upper rail or cover. ☐ ☐

7. Pull the clean sheet across the crib and miter or fit the corners. ☐ ☐

8. Adjust the crib bumpers if they are used. ☐ ☐

Note: Never use a pillow in an infant's crib because he may suffocate. ☐ ☐

9. Place the infant back into the crib. Cover him with the baby blanket if he will be sleeping.

10. Raise the side rail and pull the upper rail or cover into position. ☐ ☐

Completion

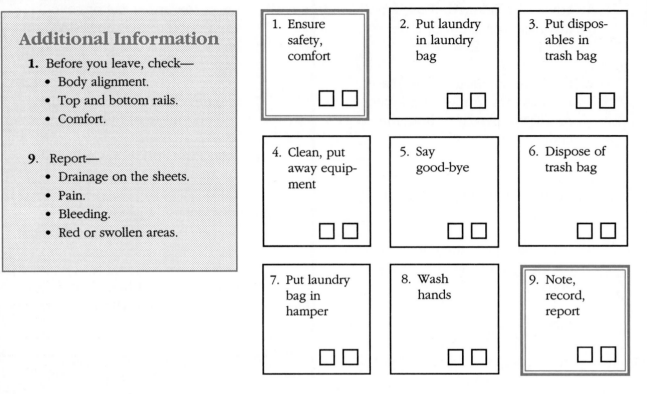

1. Ensure safety, comfort ☐ ☐

2. Put laundry in laundry bag ☐ ☐

3. Put disposables in trash bag ☐ ☐

4. Clean, put away equipment ☐ ☐

5. Say good-bye ☐ ☐

6. Dispose of trash bag ☐ ☐

7. Put laundry bag in hamper ☐ ☐

8. Wash hands ☐ ☐

9. Note, record, report ☐ ☐

_____

Student   Date

_____

Instructor   Date

Skill 38: Helping a Person Eat

Precautions

- When offering hot fluid through a straw, use caution so that the person does not burn his throat.
- Offer food slowly and in small amounts to prevent the person from choking.
- To avoid possible aspiration, make sure the person is awake and alert before offering food or drink.
- Check the person's diet before offering food.

Preparation

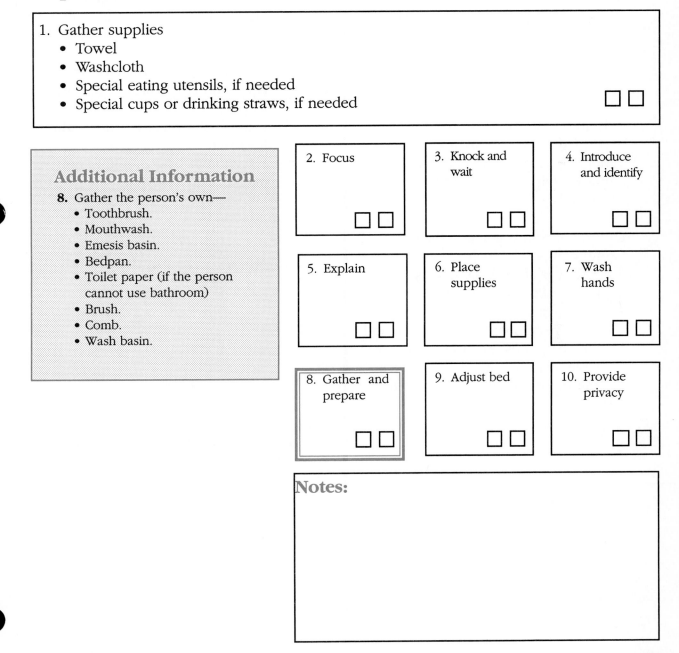

1. Gather supplies
   - Towel
   - Washcloth
   - Special eating utensils, if needed
   - Special cups or drinking straws, if needed

Additional Information

8. Gather the person's own—
- Toothbrush.
- Mouthwash.
- Emesis basin.
- Bedpan.
- Toilet paper (if the person cannot use bathroom)
- Brush.
- Comb.
- Wash basin.

2. Focus

3. Knock and wait

4. Introduce and identify

5. Explain

6. Place supplies

7. Wash hands

8. Gather and prepare

9. Adjust bed

10. Provide privacy

Notes:

Procedure

Three tasks for helping a person eat are—

1. Preparing a person for mealtime.

2. Serving a meal tray.

3. Feeding a person.

Task 1: Preparing a Person for Mealtime

1. Help the person brush her hair. □ □

2. Help her use the bathroom, bedside commode, or bedpan, as needed. Make sure the person is dressed appropriately. □ □

3. Help the person wash her hands and face. If she wears glasses or dentures, make sure they are in place. Help with oral care as needed. □ □

4. If the person is going to the dining room,—
 • Help her as necessary, to be seated at the table. Ask where she would like to sit.
 • If the person is in a wheelchair and the chair does not fit under the table, help her into a chair which can be pulled close to the table.

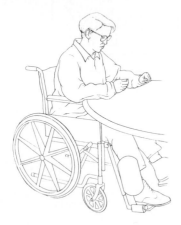

5. If the person is remaining in his room, be sure the room is well lighted. □ □

If the person can be out of bed—
 • Encourage him to sit in a chair at the bedside.

Note: If you are using a geriatric feeding chair, make sure that the wheels are locked, that the person's feet are on the footrest, and that the adjustable tray is locked securely in the tray notches.
 • Position a tray table in front of the person.
 • Place a clothing protector on his chest and lap to protect against spills.
 • Place fresh drinking water within his reach.
 • Place the call signal within his reach.

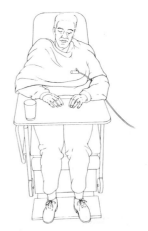

If the person cannot or chooses not to be moved from the bed—
 • Change any soiled bed linens.
 • Position the person in Fowler's position with the tray table across the bed.
 • Fluff and turn her pillow.
 • Place a clothing protector under the person's chin to protect against spills.

176

- Place fresh drinking water within her reach.
- Place the call signal within her reach.

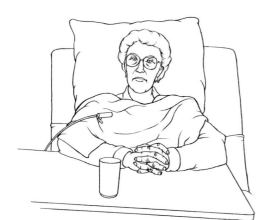

Task 2: Serving a Meal Tray

1. Bring the tray to the person. Make sure the name on the tray matches the name of the person. □ □

2. Make sure the tray of food matches the type of diet that the person is on. Look to see if any items are missing. Also check to see that hot items are hot and cold items are cold. Correct any problems with the tray. If you have any questions, check with your supervising nurse. □ □

Note: Remove items from the tray and place them directly on the table, if possible, to create a warmer atmosphere.

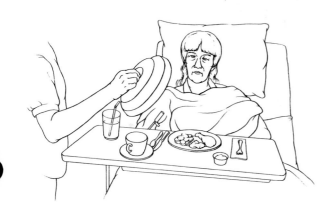

3. Hand the napkin to the person or tuck it under her chin. □ □

Note: If the person has a weak side, place the food and silverware on the person's stronger side. Use adaptive devices as needed. (Read about these in Chapter 12, Healthful Eating, in the textbook.)

4. Open any containers or packages. Butter bread and cut up food if the person needs help. If not restricted by her diet, add additional seasonings as he requests. □ □

5. Position the overbed table so that the person can easily reach the food. □ □

Task 3: Feeding a Person

1. Describe what is on the tray if the person cannot see and ask in which order he prefers to eat things.

2. Encourage the person to hold any finger foods.

3. To offer liquids by cup to a person who cannot sit upright, raise and support his head with one hand while holding the cup with the other and allowing the person to drink. □ □

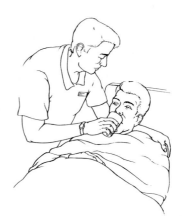

4. To offer liquids by straw, stir the liquid with the straw to distribute the heat evenly. Place the straw in the person's mouth so that she can suck and swallow the liquid as desired. (If the person sucks too much liquid, you may need to pinch off the straw and pull it away so she can swallow.) Try to avoid having the person finish all the liquid first so that she is not too full to eat the solids. ☐ ☐

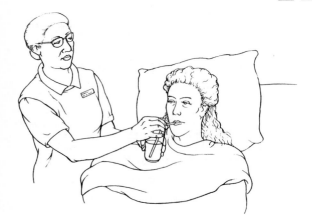

Note: Test hot liquids before serving by dropping a few drops on your wrist.

5. Feed the person slowly, naming each food as you offer it. ☐ ☐

6. Fill a spoon only two-thirds full. Touch the spoon to the person's lower lip and then to his tongue to let him know where the food is and when to open his mouth. Allow time between bites for the person to chew and swallow. Offer a liquid and then a few bites of food, followed by liquid again. ☐ ☐

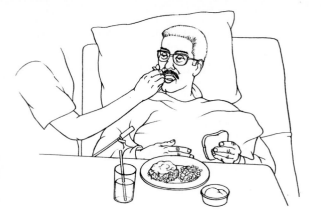

7. Wipe the person's mouth with a napkin, as needed. ☐ ☐

8. Move the tray away when the person has finished eating. ☐ ☐

Note how much the person has eaten and drunk.

9. Provide mouth care after the meal. ☐ ☐

Completion

Additional Information

1. Before you leave, check—
- Call signal.
- Body alignment.
- Bed lowered.
- Side rails, if used.
- Comfort.

4. Put on fresh gloves if there is visible blood. Clean—
- Person's things.
- Working surface.

6. Put food tray in appropriate place. In a facility, put it in the designated rack or cart. In the home, return the tray to where the dishes can be cleaned.

9. Report—
- How much the person ate and drank.
- Difficulties in eating or swallowing.

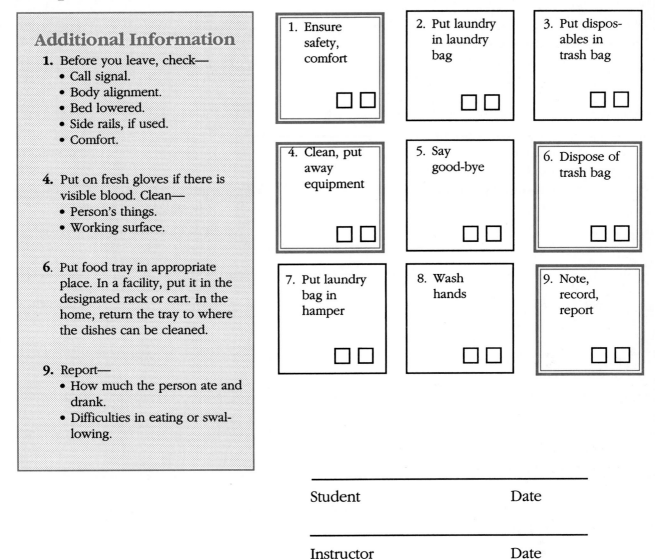

1. Ensure safety, comfort ☐ ☐	2. Put laundry in laundry bag ☐ ☐	3. Put disposables in trash bag ☐ ☐
4. Clean, put away equipment ☐ ☐	5. Say good-bye ☐ ☐	6. Dispose of trash bag ☐ ☐
7. Put laundry bag in hamper ☐ ☐	8. Wash hands ☐ ☐	9. Note, record, report ☐ ☐

_____

Student   Date

_____

Instructor   Date

Skill 39: Measuring a Person's Height and Weight

Precautions

- Use proper body mechanics.

Preparation

1. Gather supplies
   - Appropriate scales to weigh the person
   - Tape measure, if needed.
   - Paper towel
   - Towel (optional)
   - Chair (optional)

   ☐ ☐

Additional Information

8. If the person is unable to stand on his own, use a chair scale or bed scale.

2. Focus

   ☐ ☐

3. Knock and wait

   ☐ ☐

4. Introduce and identify

   ☐ ☐

5. Explain

   ☐ ☐

6. Place supplies

   ☐ ☐

7. Wash hands

   ☐ ☐

8. Gather and prepare

   ☐ ☐

9. Adjust bed

   ☐ ☐

10. Provide privacy

   ☐ ☐

Notes:

Procedure

Option 1: Measuring a Person in Bed

1. Have the person lie as flat and straight as possible. □ □

2. Using a tape measure, measure the person from the top of her head to the soles of her feet. □ □

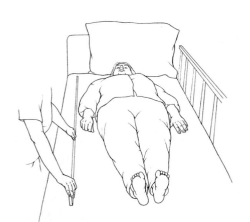

3. Write down the measurement in feet and inches. □ □

Option 2: Measuring a Person's Weight Using a Bathroom Scale

1. Help the person remove shoes and unnecessary clothing. Provide a chair for her to sit on, and a towel to stand on, if needed. □ □

2. Place a paper towel on the scale. □ □

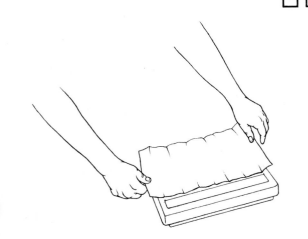

3. Help the person stand on the scale. Make sure she can stand alone safely. Always keep one hand close behind a person if he is unsteady on his feet. □ □

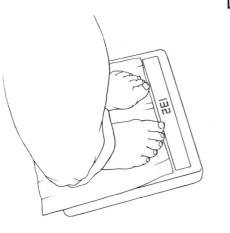

4. Read and remember the weight shown on the scale dial. □ □

5. Help the person off the scale. □ □

6. Help the person with clothing and shoes, as needed. □ □

Option 3: Measuring A Person's Height and Weight Using an Upright Scale

1. Check the balance of the scale by moving the weight all the way to the left (zero). The pointer should swing evenly between the top and bottom of the metal square. If the scale is not balanced, notify the nurse. □ □

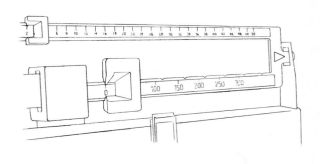

2. Put a paper towel on the scale. ☐ ☐

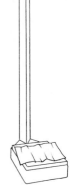

3. Help the person take off her robe and slippers. ☐ ☐

4. Help the person onto the scale platform. Make sure she can stand up on the platform without help. Always keep one hand close behind a person who is unsteady on her feet. ☐ ☐

Note: If the person is unable to stand on her own, use a chair scale or bed scale.

5. Measure the person's height. Ask her to stand up as straight as possible. Raise the measuring rod so that you can straighten the extension. Lower the measuring rod until the extension touches the top of the person's head and is level. ☐ ☐

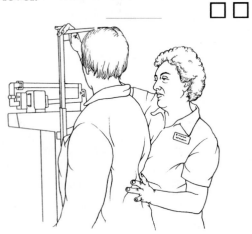

6. Move the measuring rod out of the way and write down the height measurement. ☐ ☐

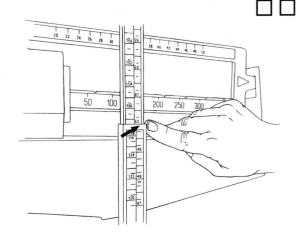

7. Measure the person's weight. Move the lower weight until the pointer drops to the bottom of the square. Move the weight backward one notch. Move the upper weight until the pointer balances. Add the two weights together and write down the sum. ☐ ☐

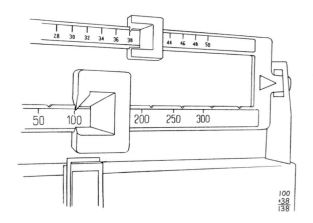

$$\begin{array}{r} 100 \\ +38 \\ \hline 138 \end{array}$$

Note: If you are using a scale designed for a person seated in a chair, subtract the chair weight from the total weight.

8. Assist the person off the scale, and help her back to her room. ☐ ☐

Completion

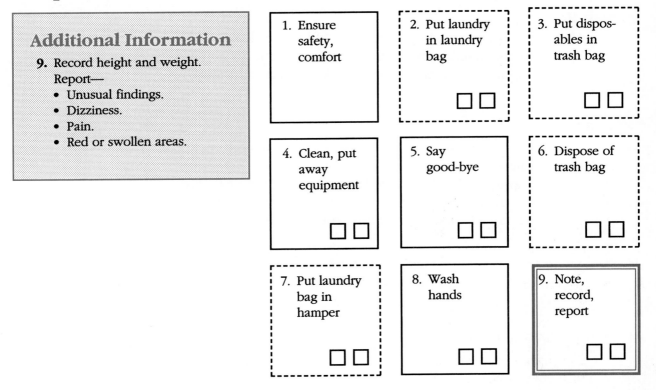

1. Ensure safety, comfort

2. Put laundry in laundry bag ☐ ☐

3. Put dispos-ables in trash bag ☐ ☐

4. Clean, put away equipment ☐ ☐

5. Say good-bye ☐ ☐

6. Dispose of trash bag ☐ ☐

7. Put laundry bag in hamper ☐ ☐

8. Wash hands ☐ ☐

9. Note, record, report ☐ ☐

_____

Student   Date

_____

Instructor   Date

Skill 40: Helping a Person Use the Bathroom Toilet

Precaution

- Make sure the person in your care is safe before leaving him alone in the bathroom door. Stay just outside the bathroom door. Check on him at least every 5 minutes to make sure he is okay and to see if he needs any assistance.

Preparation

1. Gather supplies
   - Towel and wash cloth (if you need to assist with perineal care)
   - Two pairs of disposable gloves (if you need to assist with perineal care)
   - Plastic trash bag (if you need to assist with perineal care) ☐ ☐

Additional Information

8. Gather the person's own:
- Robe.
- Slippers.

Help him put on the robe and slippers.

Why? Putting on the robe and slippers provides warmth, privacy, and safety.

If you are going to measure output, make sure a collection container is in the toilet.

2. Focus ☐ ☐	3. Knock and wait ☐ ☐	4. Introduce and identify ☐ ☐
5. Explain ☐ ☐	6. Place supplies ☐ ☐	7. Wash hands ☐ ☐
8. Gather and prepare ☐ ☐	9. Adjust bed ☐ ☐	10. Provide privacy ☐ ☐

Notes:

Procedure

1. Help the person get to the bathroom, either by walking or by moving in a wheelchair. ☐ ☐

2. Help the person adjust clothing and sit on the toilet. ☐ ☐

Note: Pay particular attention to proper body mechanics because the bathroom may be a cramped space that is difficult to move in properly, and the toilet may be low.

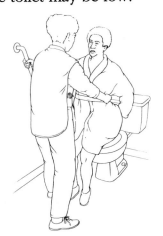

3. Make sure the toilet paper and call signal are within the person's reach. ☐ ☐

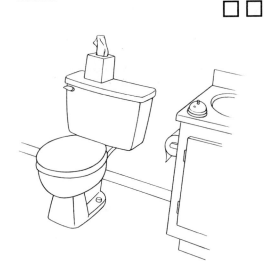

4. If a male wishes to stand while urinating, make sure he is safe if you leave him alone. ☐ ☐

5. If it is safe to leave the person alone, leave the bathroom and close the door to give the person privacy. Wait outside the door until the person has finished. ☐ ☐

6. Return to the room when the person signals. If the person cannot or does not signal, check on her at least every 5 minutes. ☐ ☐

7. Put on gloves if you need to help the person wipe with the toilet paper or to clean herself. Always clean a female from front to back. When you have finished, take off the gloves and throw them away in the plastic trash bag. ☐ ☐

8. Help the person get off the toilet. Adjust her clothing. ☐ ☐

9. Help the person use soap to wash her hands. ☐ ☐

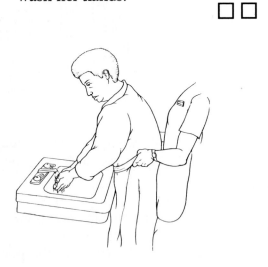

10. Help the person return to her room. If she is returning to bed, help her take off her robe and slippers. Help her back into bed. ☐ ☐

Completion

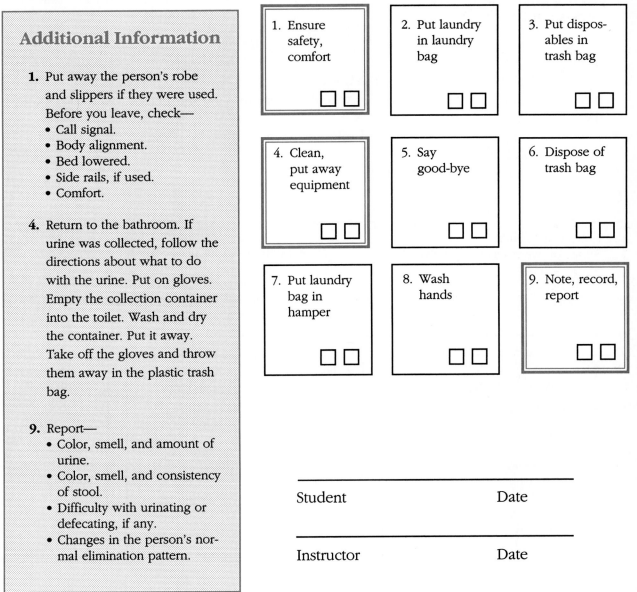

1. Ensure safety, comfort ☐ ☐

2. Put laundry in laundry bag ☐ ☐

3. Put disposables in trash bag ☐ ☐

4. Clean, put away equipment ☐ ☐

5. Say good-bye ☐ ☐

6. Dispose of trash bag ☐ ☐

7. Put laundry bag in hamper ☐ ☐

8. Wash hands ☐ ☐

9. Note, record, report ☐ ☐

_____

Student   Date

_____

Instructor   Date

187

Skill 41: Helping a Person Use a Portable Commode

Precautions

- Check with your supervising nurse before moving the person from the bed to the commode.
- Make sure the collection container is under the seat.
- If the commode has wheels, lock the wheels before moving the person from the bed to the commode.
- Check on the person at least every 5 minutes to make sure he is okay and to see if he needs any assistance.
- Ask a co-worker to help, if needed.

Preparation

1. Gather supplies
   - One or two pairs of disposable gloves
   - Plastic trash bag
   - Washcloth
   - Towel
   - Laundry bag (or plastic bag for wet or soiled laundry)
   - Collection container cover
   - Portable commode with collection container (if one is not already present in the room) ☐ ☐

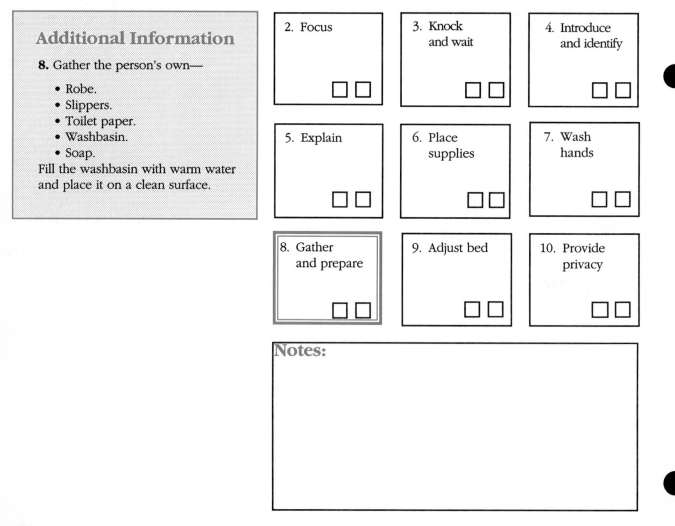

Additional Information

8. Gather the person's own—

   - Robe.
   - Slippers.
   - Toilet paper.
   - Washbasin.
   - Soap.

   Fill the washbasin with warm water and place it on a clean surface.

2. Focus ☐ ☐

3. Knock and wait ☐ ☐

4. Introduce and identify ☐ ☐

5. Explain ☐ ☐

6. Place supplies ☐ ☐

7. Wash hands ☐ ☐

8. Gather and prepare ☐ ☐

9. Adjust bed ☐ ☐

10. Provide privacy ☐ ☐

Notes:

Procedure

1. Move the portable commode to the side of the bed and place it in a way that will ensure a safe transfer of the person from the bed to the commode. You may have to place the commode against the wall for stability. Lift the lid of the commode and remove the pail cover. ☐ ☐

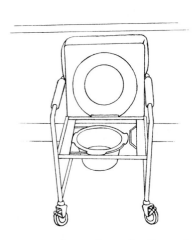

2. Lower the side rail, if used. ☐ ☐

3. Help the person sit on the side of the bed. Help her put on her robe and slippers. ☐ ☐

4. Transfer her to the commode as you would transfer her to a chair. (Review Skill 18, Transferring a Person from the Bed to a Chair.) Help her adjust her clothing as she sits on the commode.

☐ ☐

5. Make sure the toilet paper and call signal are within reach. Leave the room if it is safe to leave the person alone. Wait outside the door until the person has finished. ☐ ☐

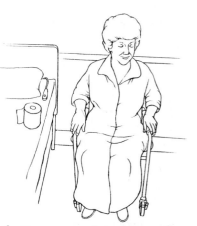

6. Return to the room when the person signals. If she cannot or does not signal, check on her at least every 5 minutes. ☐ ☐

7. If the person needs help to wipe and clean after eliminating, put on disposable gloves. Always clean females from front to back. When you have finished assisting with wiping the perineal area, take off the gloves and throw them away in the plastic trash bag.

☐ ☐

8. Help the person use the wash-cloth, soap, and towel to wash and dry her hands. □ □

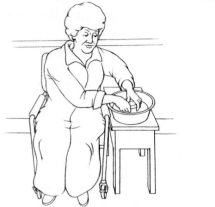

9. Using the appropriate chair-to-bed transfer, help the person get off the commode. □ □

10. Help the person back into the bed and help her take off her robe and slippers. □ □

11. Raise the side rail, if used. □ □

Completion

Additional Information

1. Before you leave, check—
   - Call signal.
   - Body alignment.
   - Bed lowered.
   - Side rails, if used.
   - Comfort.

4. Put on a new pair of disposable gloves. Remove the collection container from the commode, and cover it with the cover. Take the collection container to the dirty utility room or to the bathroom, empty it, and clean it.

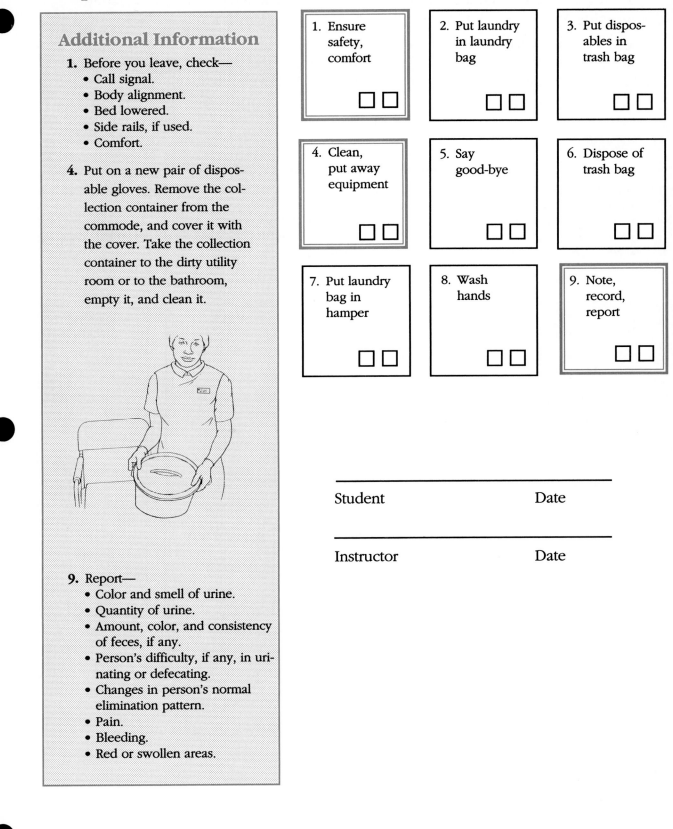

9. Report—
   - Color and smell of urine.
   - Quantity of urine.
   - Amount, color, and consistency of feces, if any.
   - Person's difficulty, if any, in urinating or defecating.
   - Changes in person's normal elimination pattern.
   - Pain.
   - Bleeding.
   - Red or swollen areas.

1. Ensure safety, comfort ☐ ☐	**2.** Put laundry in laundry bag ☐ ☐	**3.** Put disposables in trash bag ☐ ☐
4. Clean, put away equipment ☐ ☐	**5.** Say good-bye ☐ ☐	**6.** Dispose of trash bag ☐ ☐
7. Put laundry bag in hamper ☐ ☐	**8.** Wash hands ☐ ☐	**9.** Note, record, report ☐ ☐

_____

Student   Date

_____

Instructor   Date

Skill 42: Helping a Person Use a Bedpan or Urinal

Precautions

- Check a person who is sitting on the bedpan or using a urinal at least every 5 minutes to make sure he is okay or to see if he needs assistance. If the person is on the bedpan or has a urinal in place for longer than 5 minutes, he can develop pressure sores.

Preparation

1. Gather supplies
   - Disposable bed protector
   - Two pairs of disposable gloves
   - Plastic trash bag
   - Washcloth
   - Towel
   - Bedpan or urinal cover
   - Laundry bag (or plastic bag for wet or soiled laundry) ☐ ☐

Additional Information

1. Using a bedpan is not very comfortable and may feel unnatural. It is important to help the person into a position that best resembles sitting on a toilet. You could elevate the head of the bed and ask the person to bend his knees, if possible.

8. Gather the person's own—
   - Bedpan or urinal.
   - Toilet paper.
   - Washbasin.
   - Powder.
   - Soap.

2. Focus ☐ ☐	3. Knock and wait ☐ ☐	4. Introduce and identify ☐ ☐
5. Explain ☐ ☐	6. Place supplies ☐ ☐	7. Wash hands ☐ ☐
8. Gather and prepare ☐ ☐	9. Adjust bed ☐ ☐	10. Provide privacy ☐ ☐

Notes:

Procedure

1. Make sure the bedpan is dry. If the person has no open sores on the buttocks, put powder on the rim of the bedpan to make it easier to put it under the person. ☐ ☐

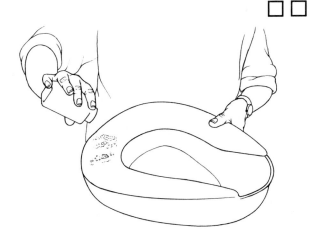

2. Lower the head of the bed so that the person is as flat as possible. ☐ ☐

3. Lower the side rail, if used, on the side where you are working. ☐ ☐

4. Fold the top linens out of the way, keeping the person's legs covered. Be sure the person's clothing is also out of the way. ☐ ☐

5. Place the disposable bed protector under the person's buttocks. ☐ ☐

For a bedpan: Help the person onto the bedpan. Ask the person to bend her knees and raise her buttocks by pushing against the mattress with her feet. Assist, as necessary, by slipping your hand under her lower back and lifting slightly.

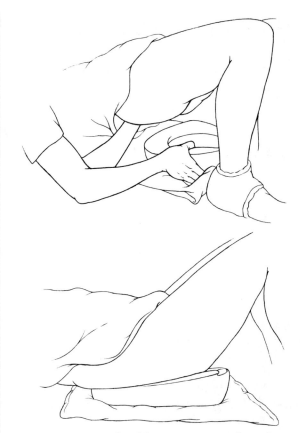

Note: Top bed linens omitted in the figure for clarify.

Note: If the person is unable to help, turn her onto her side away from you. Place the bedpan firmly against her buttocks. Gently turn the person back onto the bedpan.

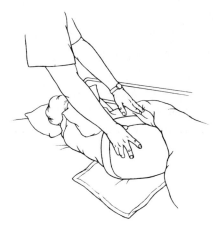

For a urinal: Give the urinal to a male. If he needs assistance, put the urinal between his legs and gently put his penis into the urinal opening.

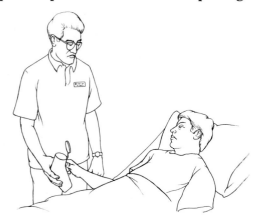

Note: It is easier and more comfortable for a male to stand while voiding. If he is not able to stand, position the urinal comfortably while he is in bed. Also, position it so that the urine will not spill.

6. Put the top linens back over the person if the person is in the bed. ☐ ☐

7. Raise the side rail, if used. Raise the head of the bed so that the person is in a comfortable sitting position. Ask her to bend her knees if possible. ☐ ☐

8. Make sure the toilet paper and call signal are within her reach. Wash your hands. Leave the room if it is safe to leave the person alone. Wait outside the door until the person has finished. ☐ ☐

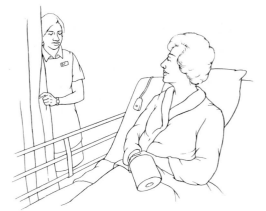

9. Return to the room when the person signals. If she cannot or does not signal, check on her at least every 5 minutes. ☐ ☐

10. When the person has finished eliminating, put on disposable gloves. ☐ ☐

11. Lower the side rail, if used. Help the person off the bedpan by having her raise her hips so that you can remove the bedpan. Or help her turn onto her side while you remove the bedpan. Set the bedpan down at the foot of the bed or place it on a nearby chair, or other suitable surface, but not on the floor or overbed table. ☐ ☐

12. Help the person wipe and clean. Provide perineal care, as necessary. Always clean a female from front to back. ☐ ☐

13. Remove the bed protector by asking the person to raise her hips again. Or, have her turn to one side while you roll the bed protector against the buttocks. Then have the person roll to the opposite side while you remove the bed protector. Throw the bed protector away in the plastic trash bag. ☐ ☐

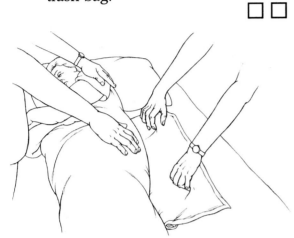

14. Take off the gloves and throw them away in the plastic trash bag. ☐ ☐

15. Help the person use the washcloth, soap, and towel to wash and dry her hands. ☐ ☐

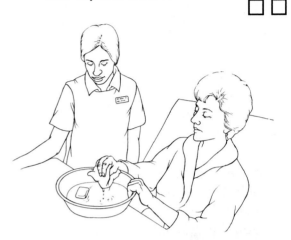

16. Help the person to a supine position. Adjust her clothing and bed linens. Raise the side rail, if used. ☐ ☐

Completion

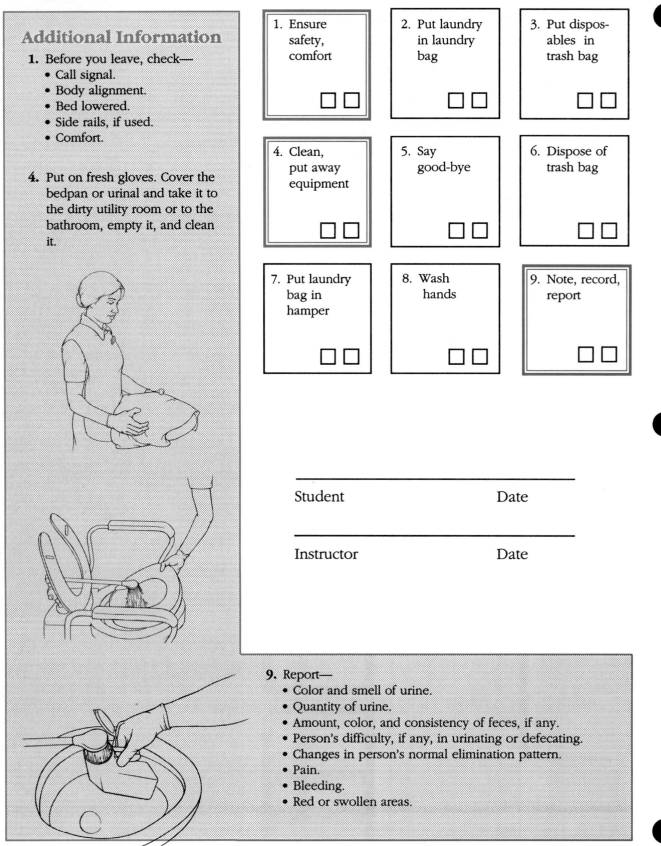

Additional Information

1. Before you leave, check—
   - Call signal.
   - Body alignment.
   - Bed lowered.
   - Side rails, if used.
   - Comfort.

4. Put on fresh gloves. Cover the bedpan or urinal and take it to the dirty utility room or to the bathroom, empty it, and clean it.

9. Report—
   - Color and smell of urine.
   - Quantity of urine.
   - Amount, color, and consistency of feces, if any.
   - Person's difficulty, if any, in urinating or defecating.
   - Changes in person's normal elimination pattern.
   - Pain.
   - Bleeding.
   - Red or swollen areas.

1. Ensure safety, comfort ☐ ☐	2. Put laundry in laundry bag ☐ ☐	3. Put disposables in trash bag ☐ ☐
4. Clean, put away equipment ☐ ☐	5. Say good-bye ☐ ☐	6. Dispose of trash bag ☐ ☐
7. Put laundry bag in hamper ☐ ☐	8. Wash hands ☐ ☐	9. Note, record, report ☐ ☐

_____

Student   Date

_____

Instructor   Date

196

Skill 43: Providing Perineal Care for a Person with a Urinary Catheter

Precautions

- Always clean the perineum from the front to the back.
- Make sure the catheter tubing is taped or secured by a fastener to the inner thigh for security.
- Make sure the drainage bag is attached to the bed and that it is lower than the person's bladder.
- Make sure the tubing is not kinked.
- Make sure the drainage bag and tubing are not touching the floor.

Preparation

1. Gather supplies
   - Bath blanket
   - Washcloth
   - Towel
   - Disposable bed protector
   - Disposable gloves
   - Paper towel
   - Plastic trash bag
   - Laundry bag (or plastic bag for wet or soiled laundry)
   - Cotton balls
   ☐ ☐

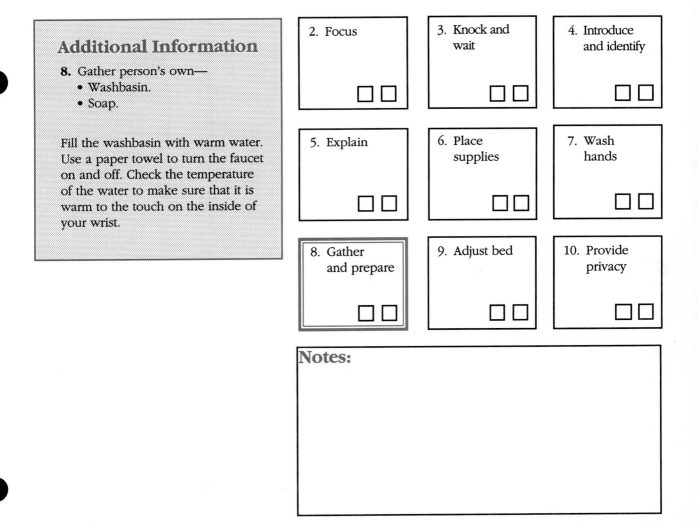

Additional Information

8. Gather person's own—
- Washbasin.
- Soap.

Fill the washbasin with warm water. Use a paper towel to turn the faucet on and off. Check the temperature of the water to make sure that it is warm to the touch on the inside of your wrist.

2. Focus ☐ ☐

3. Knock and wait ☐ ☐

4. Introduce and identify ☐ ☐

5. Explain ☐ ☐

6. Place supplies ☐ ☐

7. Wash hands ☐ ☐

8. Gather and prepare ☐ ☐

9. Adjust bed ☐ ☐

10. Provide privacy ☐ ☐

Notes:

Procedure

1. Lower the head of the bed so that the person is lying as flat as possible on her back. ☐ ☐

2. Lower the side rail, if used, on the side where you are working. ☐ ☐

3. Put the bath blanket over the person. Have the person hold the bath blanket under her chin while you fold the top covers down. ☐ ☐

4. Put a disposable bed protector under the person's buttocks. Ask her to assist by bending her knees and raising her buttocks. If the person is unable to bend her knees or raise her buttocks, turn her on her side and position the bed protector. Then roll the person back onto her back. ☐ ☐

5. Drape the person's perineal area by— ☐ ☐
   - Helping the person bend her knees and spread her legs.
   - Placing the bath blanket over the person like a diamond. Put one corner at the person's neck, a corner at each side, and one corner between her legs.
   - Wrapping each side corner around her feet. Bring each corner under and around a foot. This keeps the blanket from sliding off the person.

6. Put on the disposable gloves. ☐ ☐

7. Provide perineal care as described in Skill 24, Giving a Person a Complete Bed Bath and Shampoo. Using cotton balls, wash, rinse, and dry 4 inches of the catheter, starting where it comes out of the urethra. Observe the area around the catheter for any signs of leaking urine. Also look at her skin for any signs of infection, such as redness, swelling, pus, drainage, or crusting. ☐ ☐

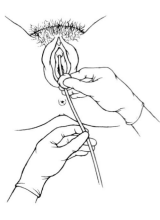

198

8. Make sure the catheter tubing is taped or secured by a fastener to the person's inner thigh for security. Allow some extra tubing so that the catheter is not being pulled. Also, make sure the bag is attached to the bed. □ □

9. Take off the gloves and throw them away in the plastic trash bag. □ □

10. Remove the disposable bed protector and throw it away in the plastic trash bag. □ □

11. Cover her with the top sheet and remove the bath blanket.

12. Raise the side rail, if used. □ □

□ □

Completion

Additional Information

1. Before you leave, check—
   - Call signal.
   - Body alignment.
   - Bed lowered.
   - Side rails, if used.
   - Comfort.

9. Record that you have completed perineal care for a person with a catheter. Report—

   - Pain.
   - Bleeding.
   - Red or swollen areas.

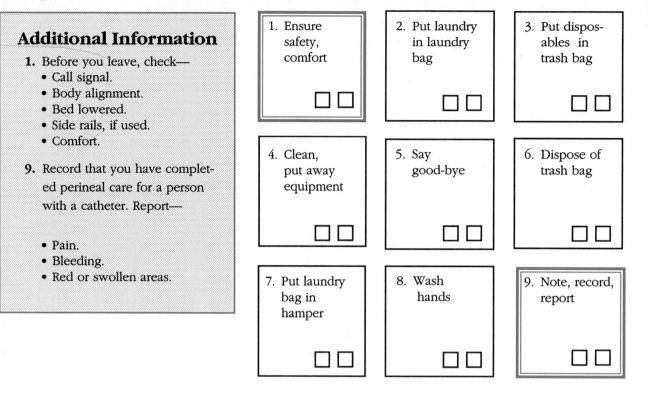

1. Ensure safety, comfort ☐ ☐

2. Put laundry in laundry bag ☐ ☐

3. Put disposables in trash bag ☐ ☐

4. Clean, put away equipment ☐ ☐

5. Say good-bye ☐ ☐

6. Dispose of trash bag ☐ ☐

7. Put laundry bag in hamper ☐ ☐

8. Wash hands ☐ ☐

9. Note, record, report ☐ ☐

_____

Student   Date

_____

Instructor   Date

Skill 44:　　　　　Urinary Drainage Bag

Precautions

- Do not allow t   ge tube to come in contact with anything except its holder.

Preparation

1. Gather supplies
   - Disposable glove
   - Graduate containe
     sure the urine (if th
     have one in the roo

   - Alcohol swab
   - Plastic trash bag

   ☐ ☐

| | 3. Knock and wait ☐ ☐ | 4. Introduce and identify ☐ ☐ |

| | 6. Place supplies ☐ ☐ | 7. Wash hands ☐ ☐ |

| 8. Gather and prepare ☐ ☐ | 9. Adjust bed ☐ ☐ | 10. Provide privacy ☐ ☐ |

Notes:

Procedure

1. Put on disposable gloves. ☐ ☐

2. Place the graduate container underneath the drain on the drainage bag. ☐ ☐

3. Remove the drain from its holder on the side of the drainage bag and open the clamp on the drain. Allow the urine to flow into the graduate. ☐ ☐

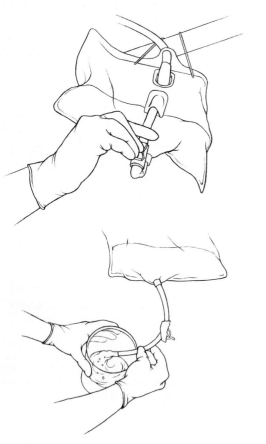

Note: The drain should not touch the graduate or the floor.

Note: Remember to use proper body mechanics as you squat to empty the urinary drainage bag.

4. Close the clamp. Wipe the end of the drainage tube with an alcohol swab. Replace the drain inside its holder. ☐ ☐

5. Take off the gloves and throw them away in the plastic trash bag. ☐ ☐

Completion

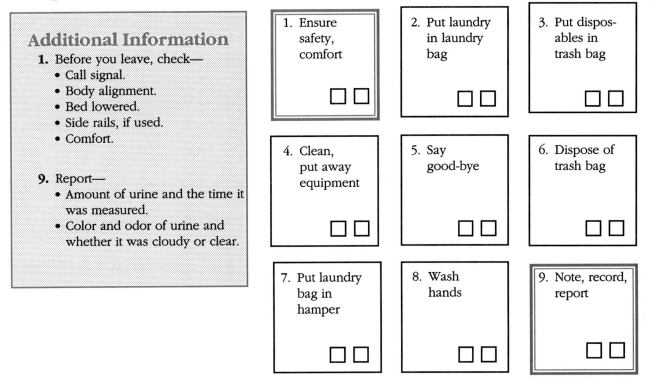

1. Ensure safety, comfort ☐ ☐

2. Put laundry in laundry bag ☐ ☐

3. Put disposables in trash bag ☐ ☐

4. Clean, put away equipment ☐ ☐

5. Say good-bye ☐ ☐

6. Dispose of trash bag ☐ ☐

7. Put laundry bag in hamper ☐ ☐

8. Wash hands ☐ ☐

9. Note, record, report ☐ ☐

_____   _____
Student   Date

_____   _____
Instructor   Date

Skill 45: Applying an External Urinary Catheter to a Male

Precautions

- Make sure the tubing does not get twisted at the tip of the man's penis.
- Check the person frequently to make sure the condom is not too tight and that there is good circulation.

Note: If you observe any swelling or color change, remove the condom and report your observations to your supervising nurse.

- When transferring the person to a chair, move the drainage bag before moving the person, and make sure the catheter is not pulled off his penis.
- Make sure the catheter tubing is taped or secured by a fastener to the person's inner thigh for security.

Preparation

1. Gather supplies
   - Bath blanket
   - External urinary catheter and drainage bag
   - Tape or catheter fastener
   - Washcloth
   - Towel
   - Bandage scissors
   - Paper towel
   - Disposable bed protector
   - Disposable gloves
   - Plastic trash bag
   - Laundry bag (or plastic bag for wet or soiled laundry) ☐ ☐

Additional Information

8. Gather the person's own—
   - Washbasin.
   - Soap.

Fill the washbasin with warm water. Use a paper towel to turn the faucet on and off. Check the temperature of the water to make sure that it is warm to the touch on the inside of your wrist.

2. Focus ☐ ☐

3. Knock and wait ☐ ☐

4. Introduce and identify ☐ ☐

5. Explain ☐ ☐

6. Place supplies ☐ ☐

7. Wash hands ☐ ☐

8. Gather and prepare ☐ ☐

9. Adjust bed ☐ ☐

10. Provide privacy ☐ ☐

Notes:

Procedure

1. Lower the side rail, if used, on the side of the bed where you are working. Put on the disposable gloves. ☐ ☐

2. Provide perineal care as described in Chapter 10, Assisting People with Personal Care, in the textbook. ☐ ☐

Why? Good perineal care should be given before applying the condom to prevent infection.

3. Put the head of the man's penis in the condom and unroll the condom over his penis. Secure the condom with the adhesive strip. Allow slack or room at the tip of his penis. ☐ ☐

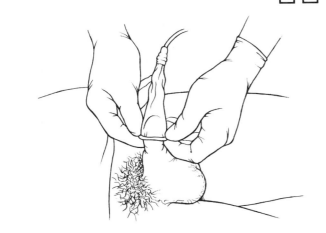

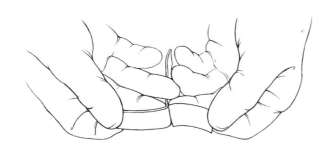

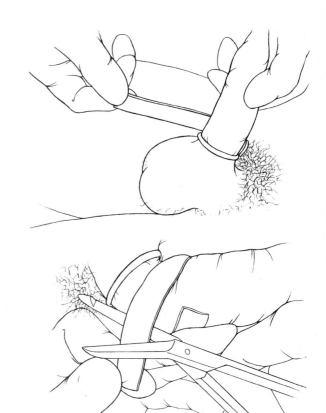

Note: Make sure the device is completely unrolled so that it does not interfere with the person's circulation.

4. Attach the condom to the drainage bag. Make sure the drainage bag is lower than the person's bladder, and hang it from the bed frame. ☐ ☐

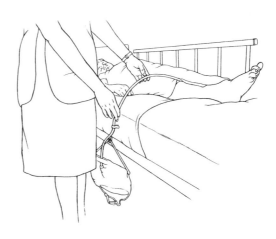

Why? For proper urine flow, the drainage bag needs to be lower than the person's bladder, but not touching the floor.

5. Use a leg band, or loosely tape the tubing to the person's inner thigh.

☐ ☐

Note: Allow some extra tubing so that the catheter is not being pulled.

6. Remove the disposable bed protector and throw it away in the plastic trash bag.

☐ ☐

7. Take off the gloves and throw them away in the plastic trash bag.

☐ ☐

8. Cover the person with the top sheet and remove the bath blanket.

☐ ☐

9. Raise the side rail, if used.

☐ ☐

Completion

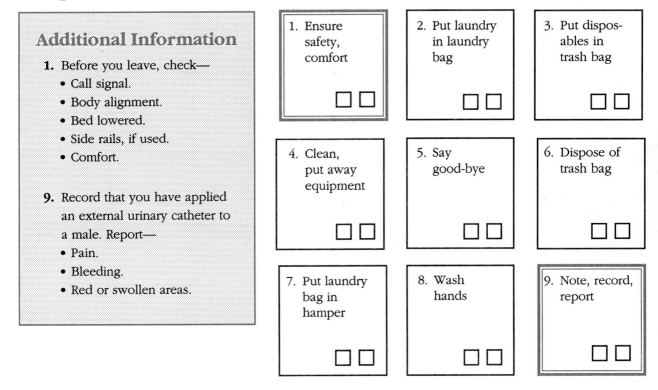

Additional Information

1. Before you leave, check—
  • Call signal.
  • Body alignment.
  • Bed lowered.
  • Side rails, if used.
  • Comfort.

9. Record that you have applied an external urinary catheter to a male. Report—
  • Pain.
  • Bleeding.
  • Red or swollen areas.

1. Ensure safety, comfort

2. Put laundry in laundry bag

3. Put disposables in trash bag

4. Clean, put away equipment

5. Say good-bye

6. Dispose of trash bag

7. Put laundry bag in hamper

8. Wash hands

9. Note, record, report

_____

Student   Date

_____

Instructor   Date

Skill 46: Collecting Urine Specimens

This skill includes three methods of collecting urine specimens: a routine urine collection; a clean catch, or midstream urine collection; and a 24-hour urine collection.

Precautions

- Always follow your supervising nurse's instructions for specimen collection.
- Remember the principles of infection control when collecting specimens.
- Always wear disposable gloves.

Preparation

1. Gather supplies
   - Specimen cup labeled with the person's name, the date and time of the collection, they type of specimen (urine), your name, and any additional information your employer requires
   - Disposable gloves
   - Urine collection hat, if the person uses the toilet
   - Plastic trash bags   ☐ ☐

Additional Information

1. For collecting a clean catch or midstream urine specimen, prepare—
   - Clean catch kit, or a sterile specimen cup.
   - Gauze squares.
   - Povidone-iodine solution.
   - Plastic trash bag

For collecting a 24-hour urine specimen, prepare—
   - Specimen collection container (usually a gallon jug).
   - Appropriate preservatives, if they are to be used.
   - Plastic trash bag.
   - Cover for bedpan, urinal, or commode container.
   - Signs.
   - Pen.
   - Tape.

8. Gather the person's own—
   - Portable commode, bedpan, or urinal.
   - Toilet paper.
   - Basin.
   - Soap.

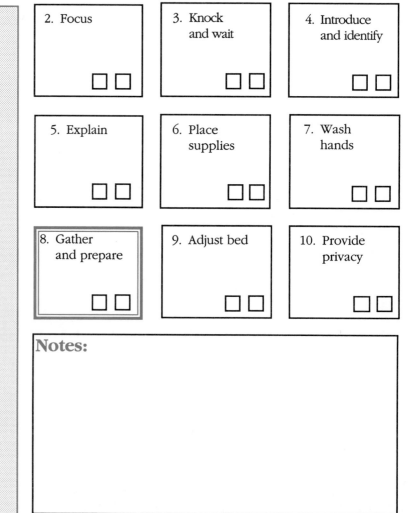

2. Focus   ☐ ☐

3. Knock and wait   ☐ ☐

4. Introduce and identify   ☐ ☐

5. Explain   ☐ ☐

6. Place supplies   ☐ ☐

7. Wash hands   ☐ ☐

8. Gather and prepare   ☐ ☐

9. Adjust bed   ☐ ☐

10. Provide privacy   ☐ ☐

Notes:

Procedure

Method 1: Routine Urine Specimen Collection

1. Following the procedure for using the bathroom toilet, portable commode, bedpan, or urinal, help the person void. ☐ ☐

   Using the bathroom toilet. Make sure there is a collection container for the person to use. This may be a specimen cup with a lid or a urine collection "hat" that sits on the rim of the toilet. If a collection hat is used, tell the person not to throw the toilet paper in the hat.

   Using a portable commode. Ask the person not to have a bowel movement and not to put the toilet paper in the commode. Put the disposable bag at the bedside for the used toilet paper.

   Using a bedpan. Do not powder the bedpan. Ask the person not to have a bowel movement and not to put the toilet paper in the bedpan. Put the disposable bag at the bedside for the used toilet paper.

   Using a urinal. No special considerations are necessary.

2. Once you have obtained the specimen in the collection container, put on disposable gloves. Take the bedpan, commode container, or urinal to the bathroom or dirty utility room. ☐ ☐

3. Pour about 60 cc of the urine into the labeled specimen cup. ☐ ☐

4. Place the lid on it. ☐ ☐

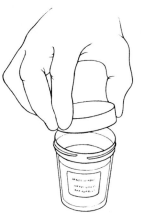

5. Take off the gloves and throw them away in the plastic trash bag. ☐ ☐

6. After you have completed the procedure for helping the person eliminate, put the cup in the designated area in the nurse's station, refrigerator, or special tray. ☐ ☐

Method 2: Clean Catch, or Midstream, Urine Specimen Collection

1. Open the clean catch kit and put it on a clean surface.

2. Offer the person an opportunity to provide his own perineal care and to collect the urine specimen without assistance. Explain the procedure. Instruct the person to—
   - Cleanse the perineal area with soap and water. Wipe the area three times with cleansing wipes in the package or with gauze squares soaked with povidone-iodine.
   - (For males) Cleanse the tip of the penis. (For uncircumcised males, retract the foreskin and keep it retracted.) Cleanse the tip of the penis with soap and water, and wipe three times with cleansing wipes or gauze squares soaked in povidone-iodine, moving in a circular pattern from the urethral opening outward, using a separate pad each time.

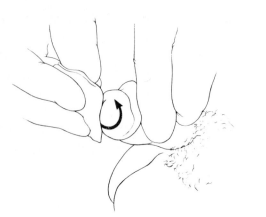

- (For females) Cleanse the labia, urethral opening, and vaginal area with cleansing wipes or gauze squares soaked in povidone-iodine. Separate the labial folds with the thumb and forefinger of one hand. Wipe down one side with a second wipe or gauze square. Throw the wipe or gauze square into a plastic trash bag. Wipe down the center with a third wipe or gauze square. Throw away wipe or gauze square in a plastic trash bag. Then wipe down the other side with a clean wipe or gauze square and throw it into a plastic trash bag. Always wipe from front to back.

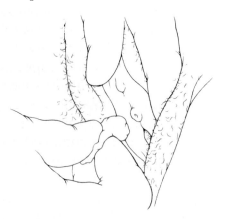

Begin voiding and then stop long enough to place a sterile container under the stream to collect midstream urine. To keep the urine clean, separate the labia or keep the foreskin retracted to protect the clean urethral opening.

Why? The initial flow of urine washes away bacteria around the urethral opening. The midstream flow will give a more accurate indication of the person's condition.

- Fill the container, remove it, and then finish voiding into the toilet, portable commode, bedpan, or urinal.

Note: It is important to return the foreskin after voiding.

Note: Stress the importance of not touching the inside of the container.

Why? Touching the inside of the container contaminates it and affects the results of the lab test. ☐ ☐

3. If the person is unable to collect the specimen, put on disposable gloves and follow the above steps to collect the specimen.

Why? Wearing gloves provides infection control.

4. After the person has finished voiding, cover the container. Do not touch the inside of the container. ☐ ☐

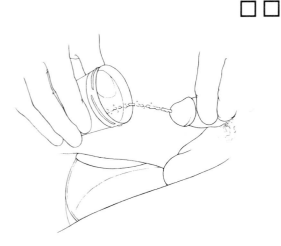

Continue to help the person with his elimination needs if necessary. Remember to record that you have completed collecting a clean catch urine specimen. Note any important observations. Note if the person had difficulty urinating. Report anything unusual to your supervising nurse.

Method 3: 24-Hour Urine Specimen Collection

1. Explain to the person that you would like to begin a 24-hour urine collection. Tell him that, for the next 24 hours, you will need him to use the toilet with a collection "hat" or use the portable commode, bedpan, or urinal so that you can collect his urine. ☐ ☐

2. Before beginning to collect urine in the specimen collection container, offer the bedpan to the person. Follow the procedure for helping a person use a bedpan. When the person has finished, discard this specimen. ☐ ☐

3. Note the time that the person voided. The time you write down is the time the collection starts. ☐ ☐

4. Prepare signs with the person's name, indicating that the person is having a 24-hour urine collection. Mark clearly on the sign the date and time that the collection started and the date and time it will end. Put the signs in all appropriate areas, such as above the person's bed or in the person's bathroom, to remind both the person and the staff that a 24-hour urine collection has started. ☐ ☐

5. Put appropriate preservatives (if they are to be used) in the specimen collection container. Check with your supervising nurse for directions. ☐ ☐

6. Have the person notify you immediately each time he voids in the collection hat, portable commode, bedpan, or urinal so that you can empty the urine into the specimen collection container. ☐ ☐

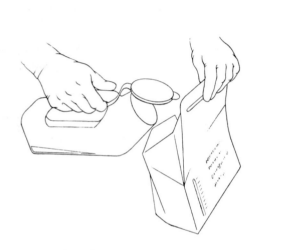

7. Have the person void at the end of the 24 hours. Add this to the container. Tell the person this is the last collection for the 24-hour period. Remove all signs about the 24-hour collection. ☐ ☐

8. Put the specimen in the designated area in the nurses' station, refrigerator, or special tray. ☐ ☐

Completion

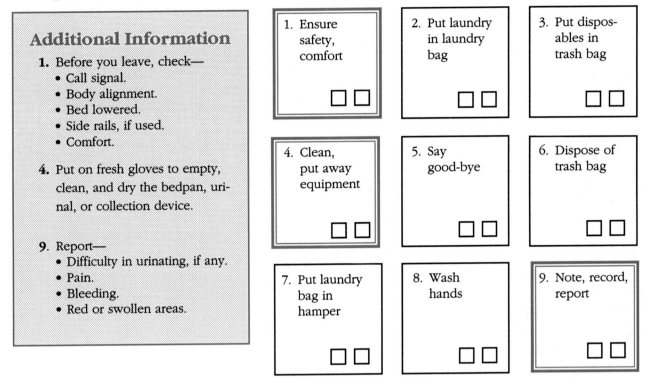

Additional Information

1. Before you leave, check—
   - Call signal.
   - Body alignment.
   - Bed lowered.
   - Side rails, if used.
   - Comfort.

4. Put on fresh gloves to empty, clean, and dry the bedpan, urinal, or collection device.

9. Report—
   - Difficulty in urinating, if any.
   - Pain.
   - Bleeding.
   - Red or swollen areas.

1. Ensure safety, comfort	☐ ☐
2. Put laundry in laundry bag	☐ ☐
3. Put disposables in trash bag	☐ ☐
4. Clean, put away equipment	☐ ☐
5. Say good-bye	☐ ☐
6. Dispose of trash bag	☐ ☐
7. Put laundry bag in hamper	☐ ☐
8. Wash hands	☐ ☐
9. Note, record, report	☐ ☐

_____
Student   Date

_____
Instructor   Date

Skill 47: Testing Urine for Sugar and Acetone

Precautions

- Always follow your supervising nurse's instructions for specimen collection.
- Remember the principles of infection control when collecting specimens.
- Always wear disposable gloves.

Preparation

1. Gather supplies
- Clinitest kit (test tube, dropper, Clinitest and Acetest tablets), Labstix, or Tes-tape
- Disposable gloves
- Paper towel
- Watch with a second hand

☐ ☐

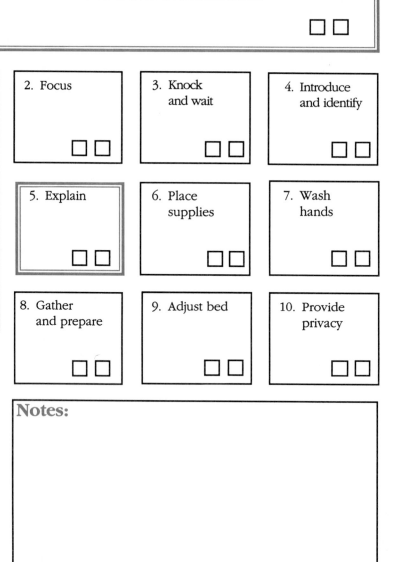

Additional Information

1. Follow the procedure and completion steps for collecting a routine urine specimen.

5. Explain to the person that you would like to test his urine for sugar and acetone. Explain that you need him to empty his bladder now and that you will be back in 1 hour to collect another specimen for the test.

2. Focus ☐ ☐

3. Knock and wait ☐ ☐

4. Introduce and identify ☐ ☐

5. Explain ☐ ☐

6. Place supplies ☐ ☐

7. Wash hands ☐ ☐

8. Gather and prepare ☐ ☐

9. Adjust bed ☐ ☐

10. Provide privacy ☐ ☐

Notes:

Procedure

This skill includes three methods for testing urine for sugar and acetone:
- Using Clinitest tablets
- Using Labstix
- Using Tes-tape

Method 1: Procedure for Using Clinitest and Acetest Tablets

1. Put on disposable gloves. ☐ ☐

2. Collect a urine specimen from the person. Take it to the dirty utility room or bathroom. ☐ ☐

3. Hold the test tube between your thumb and forefinger near the top or place it in a test tube rack. ☐ ☐

Note: Always hold the test tube at the top, because the bottom of the test tube becomes very hot to touch after the Clinitest tablet is put into the solution.

4. Fill the dropper with cold water from the running faucet. ☐ ☐

5. Holding the dropper upright over the test tube, and drop 10 drops of water into the tube. ☐ ☐

6. Empty the water from the dropper and fill it with urine from the specimen, and drop 5 drops of urine into the tube with the water. ☐ ☐

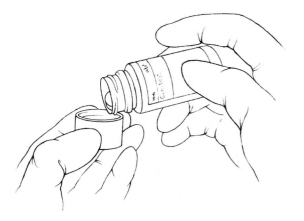

7. Dispense one tablet into the lid of the jar, and drop it into the test tube without touching it. ☐ ☐

Note: Touching the Clinitest tablet with your hands could affect the accuracy of the test.

8. Hold the tube still as you wait 15 seconds while the solution boils. ☐ ☐

Why? Holding the test tube still prevents changes to the test results.

215

9. After the solution stops boiling, shake the tube gently and check the color of the solution against the Clinitest color chart. Write down the reading. □ □

10. Put an Acetest tablet on the paper towel without touching the tablet. To do this, shake out one tablet into the lid of the jar, and drop it onto the paper towel. □ □

11. Put one drop of urine from the dropper on the Acetest tablet and wait 30 seconds. □ □

12. Check the color of the Acetest tablet against the color chart. Write down the reading. □ □

13. Discard the urine specimen if it is not needed for another test. □ □

14. Continue wearing the gloves while cleaning the equipment that has been in contact with the person's urine. □ □

Method 2: Procedure for Using Labstix

1. Remove a test strip from the bottle and recap the bottle. Hold the end of the strip with the pads in the urine for 2 seconds and then remove it. Before the test, the pad for acetone is buff colored and the glucose pad is blue. □ □

2. Remove the strip and hold it horizontally. Wait 15 seconds before comparing the color of the strip with the color on the Labstix color chart. Write down the acetone result after 15 seconds and the glucose result after 30 seconds. □ □

3. Discard the urine specimen if it is not needed for another test. ☐ ☐

4. Continue wearing the gloves while cleaning the equipment that has been in contact with the person's urine. ☐ ☐

Method 3: Procedure for Using Tes-tape

1. Remove a strip of Tes-tape about 4 inches long from the roll. ☐ ☐

2. Dip one end of the strip into the urine and remove it. ☐ ☐

3. After waiting 60 seconds, compare the darkest color of the tape with the Tes-tape color chart. Write down the reading. ☐ ☐

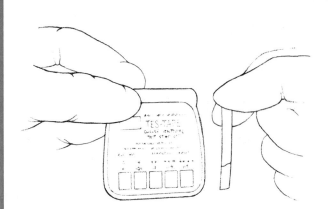

4. Discard the urine specimen if it is not needed for another test. ☐ ☐

5. Continue wearing the gloves while cleaning the equipment that has been in contact with the person's urine. ☐ ☐

Completion

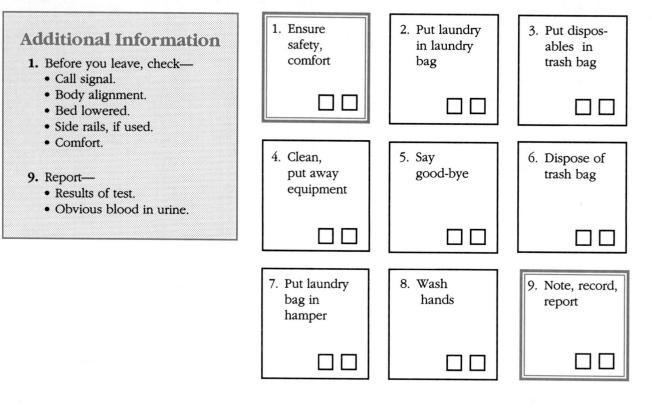

1. Ensure safety, comfort ☐ ☐

2. Put laundry in laundry bag ☐ ☐

3. Put disposables in trash bag ☐ ☐

4. Clean, put away equipment ☐ ☐

5. Say good-bye ☐ ☐

6. Dispose of trash bag ☐ ☐

7. Put laundry bag in hamper ☐ ☐

8. Wash hands ☐ ☐

9. Note, record, report ☐ ☐

_____

Student   Date

_____

Instructor   Date

Skill 48: Giving a Person a Tap Water or Soap Solution Enema

Precautions

- If the person complains of pain when you are giving an enema, stop the procedure and wait until the pain goes away. Reassure the person and have him take deep breaths. If the pain continues, stop and report the situation to your supervising nurse.
- Take care when putting the tip of the enema container or enema tubing into the person's rectum because rectal tissue is very delicate. Put the enema tip in only 2 to 4 inches.
- If you have difficulty putting the tip of the enema tubing at least 2 inches in the person's rectum, tell your supervising nurse.

Preparation

1. Gather supplies
   - Disposable bed protector
   - Enema unit
   - Lubricant jelly
   - Bath thermometer
   - Three pairs of disposable gloves
   - Plastic trash bag
   - Laundry bag (or plastic bag for wet or soiled laundry)
   - Bedpan cover
   - Washcloth
   - Towel
   □ □

Additional Information

8. Gather the person's own—
   - Bedpan.
   - Toilet paper.
   - Washbasin.
   - Soap.
   - Prepare the enema solution by clamping the tubing and filling the enema container with the amount of water ordered by the doctor.

Note: The usual amount is 500 to 1000 cc of warm water (105° Fahrenheit).
   - Test the temperature of the water to make sure it is not too hot or too cold. Use a bath thermometer to test the water temperature tosee if it si 105° Fahrenheit. If you are giving a soap suds enema, empty the mild liquid soap packet into the filled enema container.

Note: Do not agitate the soap, as soap bubbles will make air enter the rectum and cause pain.
   - Unclamp the tubing and let the solution fill the tubing to get rid of the air in it. Reclamp the tubing.

2. Focus
□ □

3. Knock and wait
□ □

4. Introduce and identify
□ □

5. Explain
□ □

6. Place supplies
□ □

7. Wash hands
□ □

8. Gather and prepare
□ □

9. Adjust bed
□ □

10. Provide privacy
□ □

Notes:

Procedure

1. Lower the head of the bed so that the person is as flat as is comfortable. ☐☐

2. Lower the side rail, if used, on the side where you are working. ☐☐

3. Cover the person with a bath blanket, and fold the top linens to the foot of the bed. Help the person remove her pajama bottoms or underwear, as appropriate. ☐☐

4. Help the person turn onto herleft side with her right knee bent. ☐☐

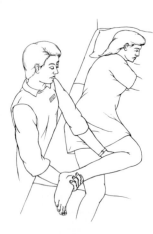

Note: Because of the way the intestine loops inside the abdomen, left-side positioning promotes the flow of the solution.

5. Place the disposable bed protector under the person's buttocks. ☐☐

6. Put the bedpan within easy reach. ☐☐

7. Put on disposable gloves. ☐☐

8. Turn back the bath blanket so that only the person's buttocks are exposed. ☐☐

9. Tear off a piece of toilet paper. Squeeze a small amount of lubricating jelly onto the toilet paper. ☐☐

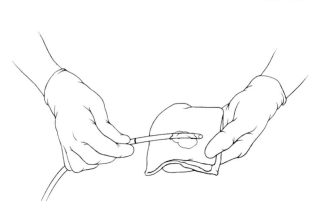

10. Lubricate the tip (2 to 4 inches) of the tubing by rotating the tip in the lubricant jelly on the paper. ☐☐

11. Raise the person's upper buttock so that her anal area shows. Gently put the enema tip into her rectum. Insert the tip no more than 2 to 4 inches. ☐☐

Note: There is a black guideline on most enema tubing to indicate the right length to insert.

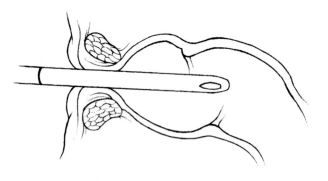

12. Tell the person to take deep breaths to relax the abdomen. ☐☐

13. Open the clamp and hold the bag or container no higher than 12 inches above his anus. ☐ ☐

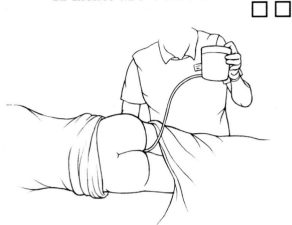

14. Allow the solution to flow slowly into the person's rectum. ☐ ☐

Note: If the person complains of cramplike pain, stop the enema until the pain goes away. Reassure the person and have her take deep breaths to relax. If she still has pain, stop the procedure and report the situation to your supervising nurse.

15. Remove the tube from the person's rectum and encourage her to hold the solution in for as long as possible. The person will retain the enema for a longer period of time if she remains in the left side-lying position. ☐ ☐

To give the person privacy, leave the room, if it is safe.

16. Help the person onto the bedpan. Make sure the toilet paper and call signal are within her reach. Raise the side rail, if used. Raise the head of the bed to a semi-Fowler's position, if possible. ☐ ☐

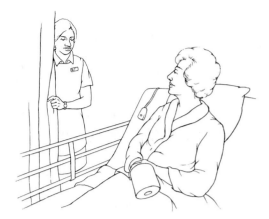

17. Remove gloves, throw them away in the plastic trash bag, and wash your hands. ☐ ☐

18. Return to the room when the person signals. If the person cannot or does not signal, check on him at least every 5 minutes. ☐ ☐

19. When the person has finished eliminating, wash your hands and fill the washbasin with warm water. Put on disposable gloves. ☐ ☐

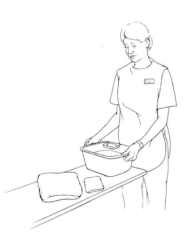

20. Lower the head of the bed and lower the side rail, if used. ☐ ☐

21. Help the person off the bedpan, and set the bedpan at the foot of the bed or on a nearby chair, or other suitable surface, but not on the floor or overbed table. ☐ ☐

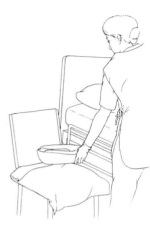

22. If needed, help the person wipe and clean. Always clean from front to back on a female. ☐ ☐

23. Remove the bed protector and throw it away in the plastic trash bag. ☐ ☐

24. Take off the gloves and throw them away in the plastic trash bag. ☐ ☐

25. Help the person put on clothing and wash her hands. Raise the side rail, if used. ☐ ☐

Completion

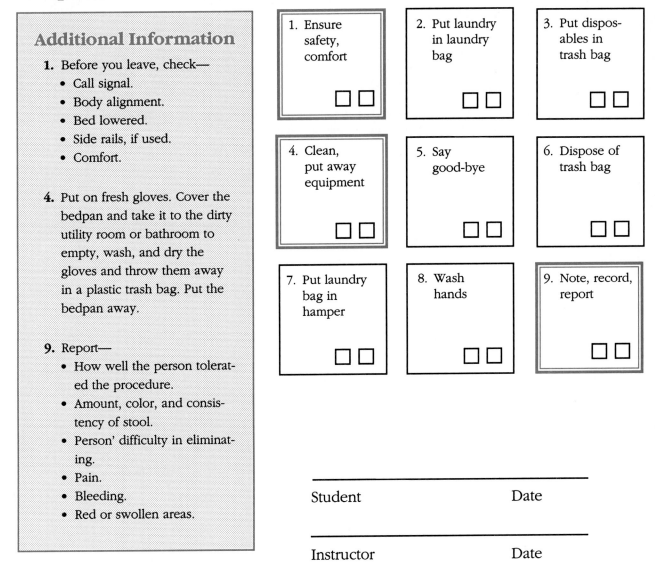

Additional Information

1. Before you leave, check—
   - Call signal.
   - Body alignment.
   - Bed lowered.
   - Side rails, if used.
   - Comfort.

4. Put on fresh gloves. Cover the bedpan and take it to the dirty utility room or bathroom to empty, wash, and dry the gloves and throw them away in a plastic trash bag. Put the bedpan away.

9. Report—
   - How well the person tolerated the procedure.
   - Amount, color, and consistency of stool.
   - Person' difficulty in eliminating.
   - Pain.
   - Bleeding.
   - Red or swollen areas.

1. Ensure safety, comfort ☐ ☐

2. Put laundry in laundry bag ☐ ☐

3. Put disposables in trash bag ☐ ☐

4. Clean, put away equipment ☐ ☐

5. Say good-bye ☐ ☐

6. Dispose of trash bag ☐ ☐

7. Put laundry bag in hamper ☐ ☐

8. Wash hands ☐ ☐

9. Note, record, report ☐ ☐

_____

Student   Date

_____

Instructor   Date

Skill 49: Giving a Person a Prepackaged Cleansing or Oil-Retention Enema

Precautions

- If the person complains of pain when you are giving an enema, stop the procedure and wait until the pain goes away. Reassure the person and have him take deep breaths. If the pain continues, stop and report the situation to your supervising nurse.
- Take care when putting the tip of the enema container or enema tubing into the person's rectum because rectal tissue is very delicate. Put the enema tip in only 2 to 4 inches.
- If you have difficulty putting the tip of the enema tubing at least 2 inches into the person's rectum, tell your supervising nurse.

Preparation

1. Gather supplies
- Disposable bed protector
- Disposable enema package
- Three pairs of disposable gloves
- Portable commode, if used
- Plastic trash bag
- Cover for bedpan or commode container
- Laundry bag (or plastic bag for wet or soiled laundry)
- Towel
- Washcloth

☐ ☐

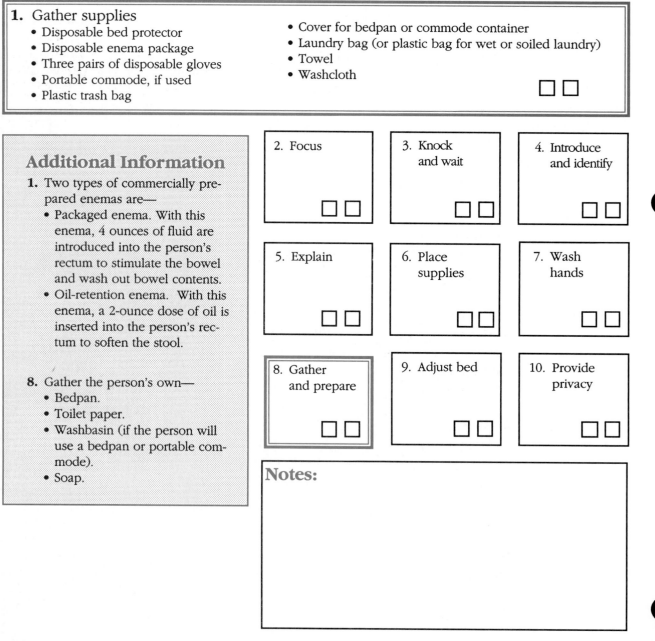

Additional Information

1. Two types of commercially prepared enemas are—
- Packaged enema. With this enema, 4 ounces of fluid are introduced into the person's rectum to stimulate the bowel and wash out bowel contents.
- Oil-retention enema. With this enema, a 2-ounce dose of oil is inserted into the person's rectum to soften the stool.

8. Gather the person's own—
- Bedpan.
- Toilet paper.
- Washbasin (if the person will use a bedpan or portable commode).
- Soap.

2. Focus ☐ ☐

3. Knock and wait ☐ ☐

4. Introduce and identify ☐ ☐

5. Explain ☐ ☐

6. Place supplies ☐ ☐

7. Wash hands ☐ ☐

8. Gather and prepare ☐ ☐

9. Adjust bed ☐ ☐

10. Provide privacy ☐ ☐

Notes:

Procedure

1. Lower the head of the bed so that the person is as flat as is comfortable. ☐ ☐

2. Lower the side rail on the side where you will be working. ☐ ☐

3. Cover the person with a bath blanket, and fold the top linens to the foot of the bed. Help the person remove her pajama bottoms or underwear, as appropriate. ☐ ☐

4. Help the person turn onto her left side with her right knee bent. ☐ ☐

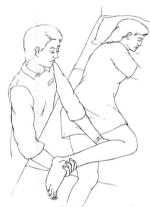

Note: Because of the way the intestine loops inside the abdomen, left-side positioning promotes the flow of the solution.

5. Place the disposable bed protector under the person's buttocks. ☐ ☐

6. Put the bedpan within easy reach. ☐ ☐

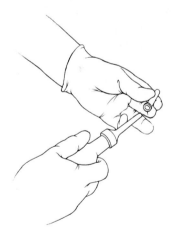

7. Put on disposable gloves. ☐ ☐

8. Turn back the bath blanket so that only the person's buttocks are exposed. ☐ ☐

9. Open the enema package and take off the protective cover. ☐ ☐

225

10. Raise the person's upper buttock so that her anal area shows. Gently put the enema tip into her rectum. Insert the tip no more than 2 to 4 inches. ☐ ☐

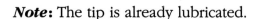

Note: The tip is already lubricated.

11. Tell the person to take deep breaths to relax the abdomen. ☐ ☐

12. Squeeze the plastic bottle slowly so that all the enema solution is given. Do not release pressure on the bottle while it is inserted in the rectum, or fluid will be drawn back into bottle from the rectum. ☐ ☐

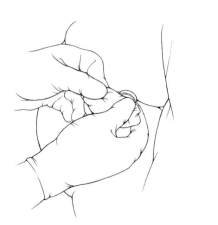

Note: If the person complains of cramplike pain, stop the enema until the pain goes away. Reassure the person and have her take deep breaths to relax. If the person still has pain, stop the procedure and report the situation to your supervising nurse.

13. Remove the tube from the person's rectum, and encourage her to hold the solution in for as long as possible. The person will retain the enema for a longer period of time if she remains in the leftside-lying position. ☐ ☐

14. Put the plastic bottle into the box to throw it away in the plastic trash bag. ☐ ☐

15. Help the person onto the bedpan, commode, or toilet. Make sure the toilet paper and call signal are within his reach. If the person is on the bedpan, raise the side rail, if used, and raise the head of the bed to a semi-Fowler's position, if possible. ☐ ☐

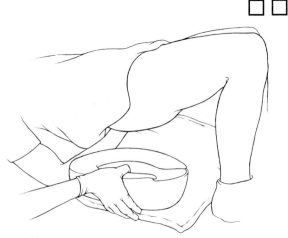

16. Take off the gloves and put them in the plastic trash bag. ☐ ☐

17. Wash your hands. To give the person privacy, leave the room if it is safe for the person to be alone. Wait outside the room until the person has finished. ☐ ☐

18. Return to the room when the person signals. If the person cannot or does not signal, check on her at least every 5 minutes. ☐ ☐

19. When the person has finished eliminating, wash your hands, fill the washbasin with warm water, and put on the disposable gloves. ☐ ☐

20. Help the person off the bedpan, and set the bedpan at the foot of the bed or on a nearby chair or other suitable surface, but not on the floor or overbed table. ☐ ☐

21. Help the person wipe and clean, as necessary. Always clean from front to back on a female. ☐ ☐

22. Remove the bed protector and throw it away in the plastic trash bag. ☐ ☐

23. Take off the gloves and throw them away in the plastic trash bag. ☐ ☐

24. Help the person off the portable commode or toilet, if used, and help her wash his hands. Help her back into bed, if she's not staying up. ☐ ☐

Completion

Additional Information

1. Before you leave, check—
- Call signal.
- Body alignment.
- Bed lowered.
- Side rails, if used.
- Comfort.

4. Put on fresh gloves. Cover the bedpan and take it to the dirty utility room or bathroom to empty, wash, and dry. Take off the gloves and throw them away in a plastic trash bag. Put the bedpan away.

9. Report—
- How well the person tolerated the procedure.
- Amount, color, and consistency of stool.
- Person's difficulty in eliminating.
- Pain.
- Bleeding.
- Red or swollen areas.

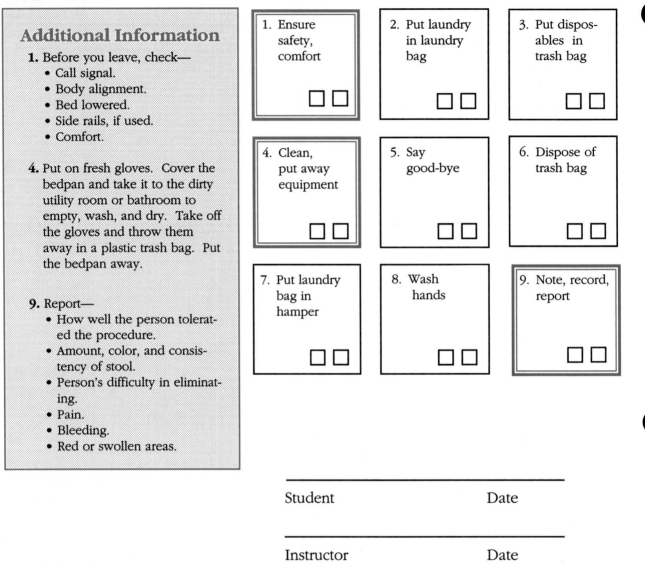

1. Ensure safety, comfort ☐ ☐

2. Put laundry in laundry bag ☐ ☐

3. Put disposables in trash bag ☐ ☐

4. Clean, put away equipment ☐ ☐

5. Say good-bye ☐ ☐

6. Dispose of trash bag ☐ ☐

7. Put laundry bag in hamper ☐ ☐

8. Wash hands ☐ ☐

9. Note, record, report ☐ ☐

_____

Student   Date

_____

Instructor   Date

Skill 50: Collecting Stool Specimens

Precautions

- Check with your supervising nurse to find out any specific instructions for collecting or handling stool specimens.
- Remember the principles of infection control when collecting specimens.
- Wear disposable gloves when handling a stool specimen.

Preparation

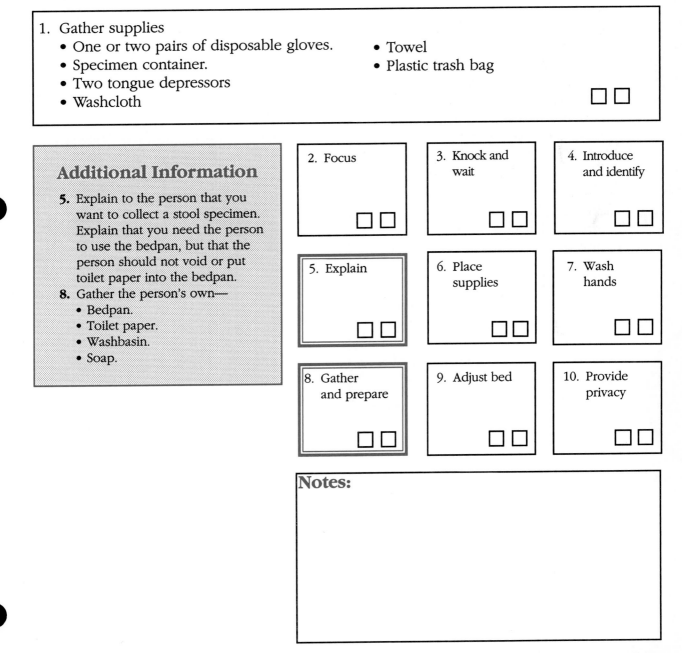

1. Gather supplies
   - One or two pairs of disposable gloves.
   - Specimen container.
   - Two tongue depressors
   - Washcloth
   - Towel
   - Plastic trash bag

   ☐ ☐

Additional Information

5. Explain to the person that you want to collect a stool specimen. Explain that you need the person to use the bedpan, but that the person should not void or put toilet paper into the bedpan.
8. Gather the person's own—
   - Bedpan.
   - Toilet paper.
   - Washbasin.
   - Soap.

2. Focus ☐ ☐

3. Knock and wait ☐ ☐

4. Introduce and identify ☐ ☐

5. Explain ☐ ☐

6. Place supplies ☐ ☐

7. Wash hands ☐ ☐

8. Gather and prepare ☐ ☐

9. Adjust bed ☐ ☐

10. Provide privacy ☐ ☐

Notes:

Procedure

Note: Have the person void first, if necessary. Put on gloves and discard the urine. Clean and dry the bedpan.

1. Lower the side rail, if used, on the side where you are working. Place the bedpan under the person's hips. Ask the person not to put toilet paper in the bedpan. Follow the procedure and completion steps for assisting with a bedpan. ☐ ☐

2. When the person has finished his bowel movement, put on disposable gloves. Remove the bedpan, cover it, and take it to the dirty utility room or to the bathroom. Take the specimen container and tongue depressor with you. Label the container with the person's name, the date, the time, specimen (stool), your name, and any additional information your employer requires, such as an ID number. ☐ ☐

3. Use the tongue depressors and remove 1 to 2 tablespoons of the stool from the bedpan and put it in the labeled container. Be careful not to contaminate the outside of the container with stool. Put the lid on the specimen container. ☐ ☐

4. Throw the tongue depressors away in the plastic trash bag. ☐ ☐

5. Empty, clean, and dry the bedpan. ☐ ☐

6. Remove the disposable gloves and throw them in the plastic tr ash bag. Wash your hand. ☐ ☐

7. Put the specimen in the designated area. If you are in a client's home, you need to follow the doctor's instructions about handling the specimen. ☐ ☐

Completion

Additional Information

1. Before you leave, check—
- Call signal.
- Body alignment.
- Bed lowered.
- Side rails, if used.
- Comfort.

9. Report—
- Color, consistency, and odor of stool.
- Person's difficulty in eliminating.
- Pain.
- Bleeding.
- Red or swollen areas.

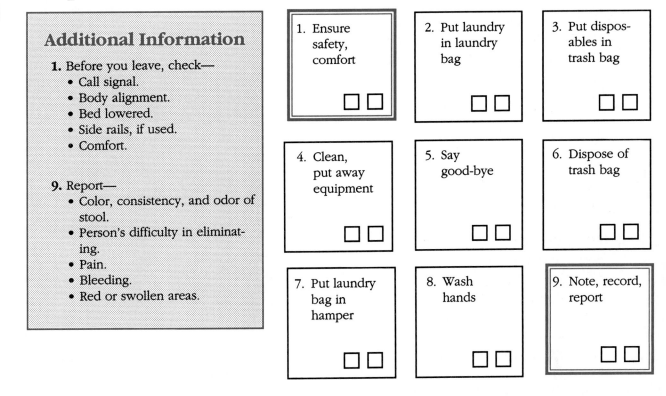

1. Ensure safety, comfort ☐ ☐

2. Put laundry in laundry bag ☐ ☐

3. Put disposables in trash bag ☐ ☐

4. Clean, put away equipment ☐ ☐

5. Say good-bye ☐ ☐

6. Dispose of trash bag ☐ ☐

7. Put laundry bag in hamper ☐ ☐

8. Wash hands ☐ ☐

9. Note, record, report ☐ ☐

_____

Student   Date

_____

Instructor   Date

Skill 51: Diapering a Child

- Always stay with the child, never leaving him alone.
- Be sure the top and bottom rails are in place if you must step away from the crib side, even if you are only turning away for a moment.

Preparation

1. Gather supplies
   - Diaper
   - Washcloth or disposable baby wipes
   - Disposable gloves
   - Towel
   - Plastic trash bag (if the room does not have a special container for disposing of soiled diapers)
   - Laundry bag (or plastic bag for wet or soiled laundry) ☐ ☐

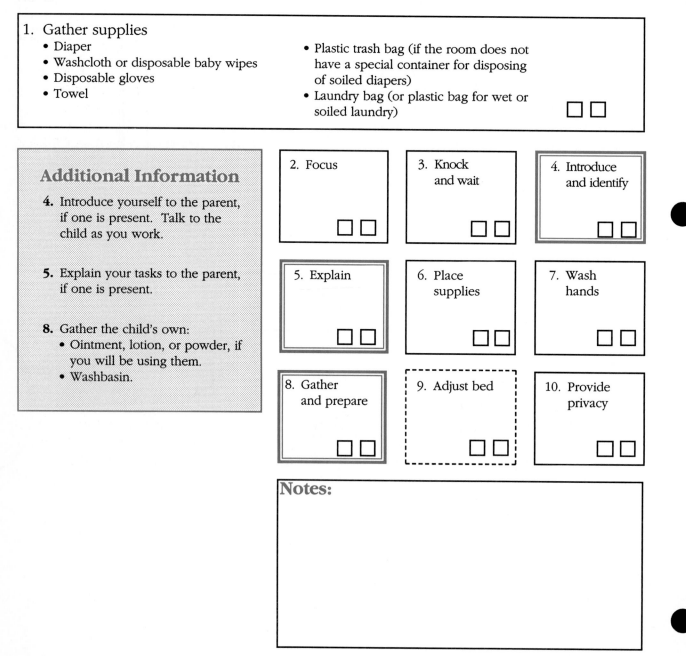

Additional Information

4. Introduce yourself to the parent, if one is present. Talk to the child as you work.

5. Explain your tasks to the parent, if one is present.

8. Gather the child's own:
   - Ointment, lotion, or powder, if you will be using them.
   - Washbasin.

2. Focus ☐ ☐

3. Knock and wait ☐ ☐

4. Introduce and identify ☐ ☐

5. Explain ☐ ☐

6. Place supplies ☐ ☐

7. Wash hands ☐ ☐

8. Gather and prepare ☐ ☐

9. Adjust bed ☐ ☐

10. Provide privacy ☐ ☐

Notes:

232

Procedure

1. Put on disposable gloves. ☐ ☐

2. Lower the crib rails. ☐ ☐

Note: If you are changing the child on a changing table, make sure all the supplies you need are within reach, so that you do not need to turn your back or walk away from the child. Pull out a clean length of paper or place a disposable pad on the changing surface.

3. Unfasten and remove the soiled diaper. If you are using pins, place them in a place where the child cannot get them. Use a clean area of the diaper to wipe feces off the child's buttocks. ☐ ☐

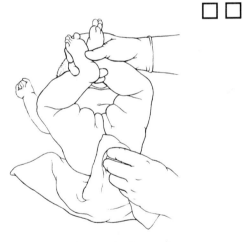

4. Use a wet washcloth or disposable wipe to clean the child's buttocks and genital areas to remove urine and feces. Wipe a female child from front to back. Pat the area dry with a towel. ☐ ☐

5. Place the soiled diaper in a plastic trash bag. If a cloth diaper is soiled with feces, roll it up so that the soiled part is to the inside and place it aside. You will need to rinse the feces from the diaper in the toilet before placing it in the diaper container. ☐ ☐

6. Apply ointment, lotion, or powder, if used. ☐ ☐

7. Put a clean diaper on the child. ☐ ☐

To put on a disposable diaper:

- Lay the diaper absorbant side up with the closure tabs at the back.
- Place the child on the diaper.
- Bring the front of the diaper up between the child's legs and fasten with the closure tabs.

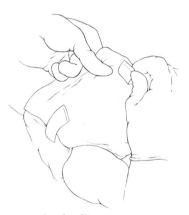

To put on a cloth diaper:

- Place the thick part of the diaper toward the back.for a female and toward the front for a male.

- Bring the front of the diaper through the child's legs and use pins to fasten. You should be able to fit two fingers between the child's abdomen and the diaper. When putting the pin through the cloth, place your fingers between the pin and the baby to help guide the pin through the cloth.

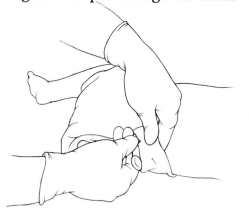

Note: Diapering the child presents a good opportunity to talk to and play with him.

8. Remove gloves and throw them in the plastic bag. ☐ ☐

9. Make sure the child's clothing is clean and dry. Change his clothing as necessary. ☐ ☐

10. Return the child to the crib and raise the side rails or put the child in another safe place. ☐ ☐

Completion

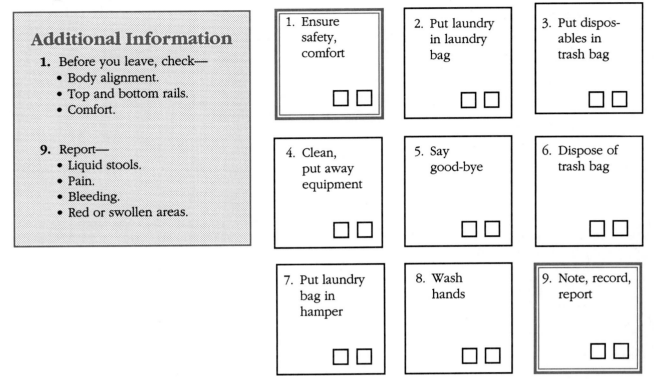

Additional Information

1. Before you leave, check—
   - Body alignment.
   - Top and bottom rails.
   - Comfort.

9. Report—
   - Liquid stools.
   - Pain.
   - Bleeding.
   - Red or swollen areas.

1. Ensure safety, comfort ☐ ☐

2. Put laundry in laundry bag ☐ ☐

3. Put disposables in trash bag ☐ ☐

4. Clean, put away equipment ☐ ☐

5. Say good-bye ☐ ☐

6. Dispose of trash bag ☐ ☐

7. Put laundry bag in hamper ☐ ☐

8. Wash hands ☐ ☐

9. Note, record, report ☐ ☐

_____
Student   Date

_____
Instructor   Date

Skill 52: Collecting a Urine Specimen from an Infant

Precautions

- Always follow your supervising nurse's instructions for urine specimen collection.
- Remember the principles of infection control when collecting specimens.
- Always wear disposable gloves.
- Always stay with the child, never leaving him alone.
- You may have to ask a co-worker to hold a very active child.

Preparation

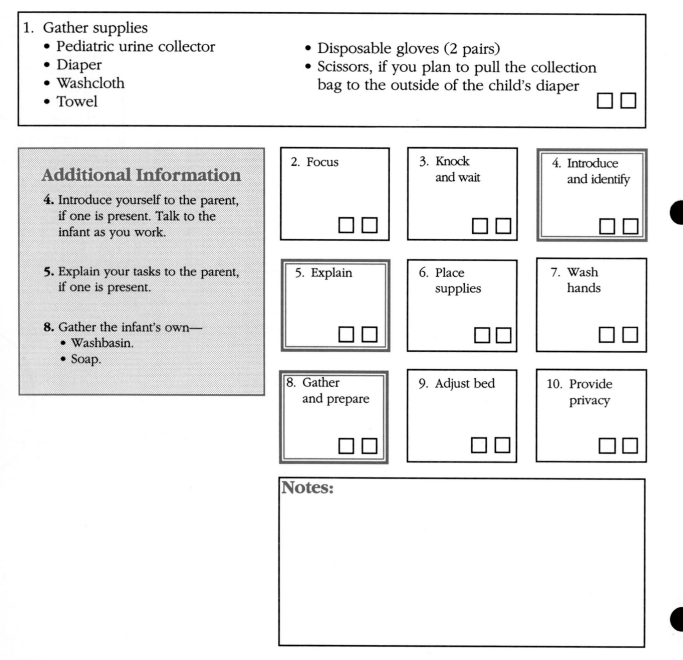

1. Gather supplies
   - Pediatric urine collector
   - Diaper
   - Washcloth
   - Towel
   - Disposable gloves (2 pairs)
   - Scissors, if you plan to pull the collection bag to the outside of the child's diaper ☐ ☐

Additional Information

4. Introduce yourself to the parent, if one is present. Talk to the infant as you work.

5. Explain your tasks to the parent, if one is present.

8. Gather the infant's own—
   - Washbasin.
   - Soap.

2. Focus ☐ ☐

3. Knock and wait ☐ ☐

4. Introduce and identify ☐ ☐

5. Explain ☐ ☐

6. Place supplies ☐ ☐

7. Wash hands ☐ ☐

8. Gather and prepare ☐ ☐

9. Adjust bed ☐ ☐

10. Provide privacy ☐ ☐

Notes:

Procedure

Obtaining a urine specimen from an infant or a child who is not toilet trained requires applying a special self-adhesive collection bag to a girl's perineal area or over a boy's penis.

1. Fill the washbasin with warm water. ☐ ☐

2. Put on disposable gloves. ☐ ☐

3. Lower the crib rail ☐ ☐

4. Remove the infant's diaper and place it in the plastic trash bag if it is wet or soiled. ☐ ☐

5. Use the washcloth, soap, and water to clean the infant's perineal area. ☐ ☐

Note: Remember that the same rules for cleaning an adult apply to the infant: clean from front to back for a female, or from the urethra outward for a male.

6. Use the washcloth to rinse. Dry the area thoroughly with a towel. ☐ ☐

7. Position the infant on his back, and spread his knees apart, exposing the genitals. (If the child is very active, you may need to ask a co-worker or the parent to hold the child.) ☐ ☐

8. Peel the sticky paper off the adhesive area at the top of the collection bag. ☐ ☐

For a male: Put his penis through the opening at the top of the bag and press the adhesive securely around the base of his penis and his scrotum.

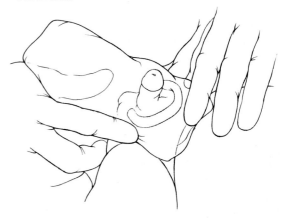

For a female: Position the bag over her urethra and press the adhesive area over her labia to create a seal.

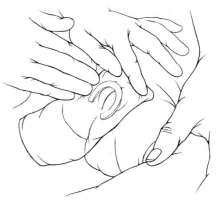

Note: Do not cover the infant's anus with the adhesive area.

9. Rediaper the infant. ☐ ☐

Note: If the infant is too young to be able to pull the bag off, you may cut a slit in the disposable diaper and pull the bag through the slit to enable you to easily see when the infant has voided.

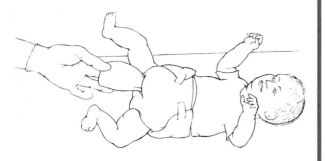

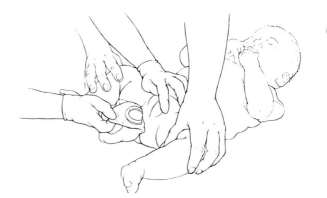

10. Remove the gloves and put them in the plastic bag. □ □

11. Raise the crib rail or put the infant in a safe place such as a playpen or infant seat. □ □

12. Empty and clean the washbasin.

13. Wash your hands and record when the bag was applied. □ □

14. Check every 15 minutes to see if the infant has urinated.

15. Wash your hands. □ □

16. After the infant has urinated, fill the washbasin with clean, warm water and take it to the cribside.

17. Put on disposable gloves. □ □

18. Lower the crib rail. □ □

19. Loosen the diaper and gently remove the bag. □ □

Seal the top by folding the adhesive area over, and place it in the sterile specimen container.

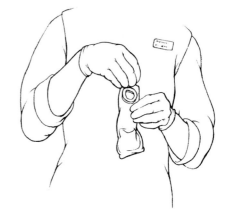

Note: Do not leave the infant unattended to do this. You may set the collection bag down on the crib and put it in the specimen container later if the infant is very active or if you cannot reach the specimen container without turning your back on the infant.

Note: Some pediatric collection bags have a port at the bottom of the bag to empty the urine into the container.

20. Clean and dry the perineal area and put a clean diaper on the infant. □ □

21. Raise the crib rail. □ □

Completion

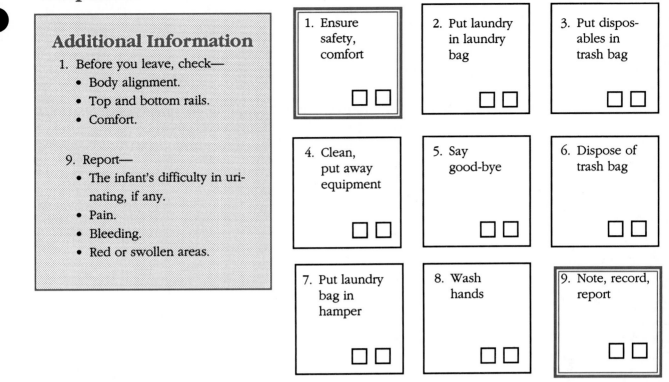

Additional Information

1. Before you leave, check—
   - Body alignment.
   - Top and bottom rails.
   - Comfort.

9. Report—
   - The infant's difficulty in urinating, if any.
   - Pain.
   - Bleeding.
   - Red or swollen areas.

1. Ensure safety, comfort ☐ ☐

2. Put laundry in laundry bag ☐ ☐

3. Put disposables in trash bag ☐ ☐

4. Clean, put away equipment ☐ ☐

5. Say good-bye ☐ ☐

6. Dispose of trash bag ☐ ☐

7. Put laundry bag in hamper ☐ ☐

8. Wash hands ☐ ☐

9. Note, record, report ☐ ☐

Student _____ Date _____

Instructor _____ Date _____

Skill 53: Helping a Person with Passive Range-of-Motion Exercises

Precautions

- Move each joint slowly, gently, and smoothly.
- Support each joint during movement.
- Always move the joint only as far as the person can tolerate it-never go beyond that point.
- Always watch the person's face, particularly his eyes, for any expression of pain. If the person has pain, stop the movement and report your observation to your supervising nurse.
- Always use proper body mechanics.

Preparation

1. Gather supplies ☐ ☐

Additional Information

9. Position the person on his back (supine position) if he can tolerate it, and make sure his body is in proper alignment.

---

2. Focus ☐ ☐	3. Knock and wait ☐ ☐	4. Introduce and identify ☐ ☐
5. Explain ☐ ☐	6. Place supplies ☐ ☐	7. Wash hands ☐ ☐
8. Gather and prepare ☐ ☐	9. Adjust bed ☐ ☐	10. Provide privacy ☐ ☐

Notes:

Procedure

The seven tasks in this procedure represent the seven sets of joints that you will exercise every time you do range-of-motion exercises for a person. They are as follows:

1. Exercising the shoulder

2. Exercising the elbow and forearm

3. Exercising the wrist

4. Exercising the fingers and thumb

5. Exercising the hip and knee

6. Exercising the ankle

7. Exercising the toes

Task 1: Exercising the Shoulder

1. Lower the side rail on the side where you are working. ☐ ☐

2. With one hand, hold the person's wrist with her palm down and put your other hand under her elbow. Provide this support throughout the following motions. ☐ ☐

3. Raise the person's arm straight up and then move it alongside her ear. Then lower the arm to her side. (The movement up toward his ear is called *flexion*. The movement down to her side is called *extension*.) Repeat five times. ☐ ☐

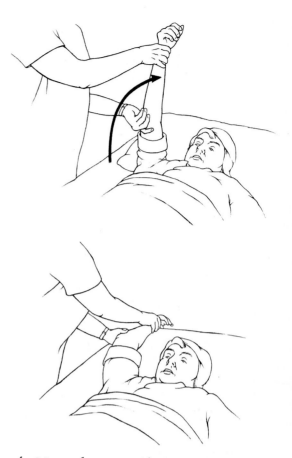

4. Move the person's arm out away from her body and return it to her side. (The movement away from the body is called *abduction*. The movement back to the body is called *adduction*.) Repeat five times. ☐ ☐

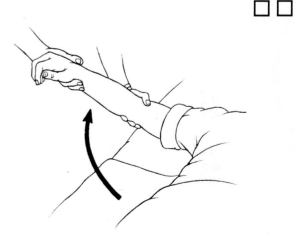

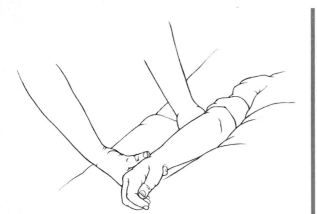

5. Carry the person's hand to the opposite shoulder, then back down to the bed. (The movement toward the shoulder is called *horizontal abduction*. The movement back to the side is called *horizontal adduction*.) ☐ ☐

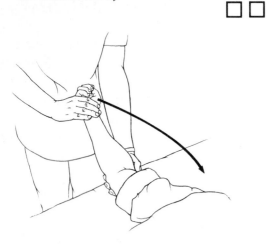

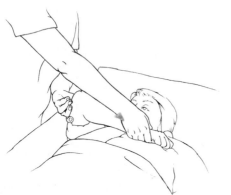

6. Raise the person's elbow so that it is at the same height as the shoulder. Move her forearm up and down, as a police officer does when signaling a person to stop. (This movement up and down is called *rotation*). Repeat five times. ☐ ☐

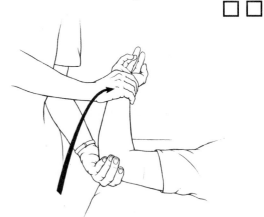

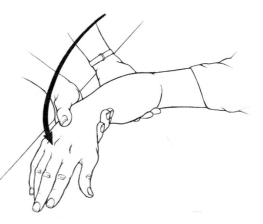

Task 2: Exercising the Elbow and Forearm

1. Hold the person's wrist with one hand and put your other hand under her elbow. Provide this support throughout the following motions. ☐ ☐

2. Bend the person's arm at the elbow so her hand moves toward her shoulder on the same side *(flexion)*. Then straighten her arm back down to the hip *(extension)*. Repeat five times. ☐ ☐

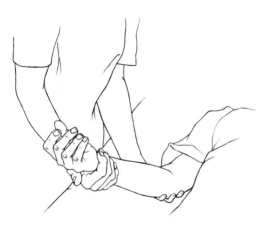

3. With the person's forearm at a right angle to the bed, turn her hand down toward her feet *(pronation)*. Then turn her hand toward her face *(supination)*. Repeat five times. ☐ ☐

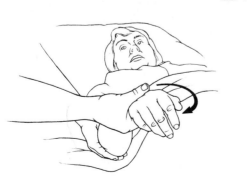

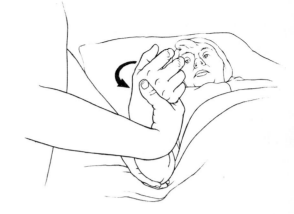

Task 3: Exercising the Wrist

1. Hold the person's wrist with one hand and her fingers with your other hand. Provide this support throughout the following motions. ☐ ☐

2. Raise her hand off the mattress. ☐ ☐

3. Move the person's hand downward *(flexion)* and then straighten the wrist *(extension)*. Move the hand back *(hyperextension)*. Repeat five times. ☐ ☐

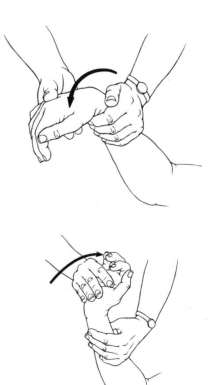

4. Straighten the wrist. Move the wrist from side to side (*abduction* and *adduction*). ☐ ☐

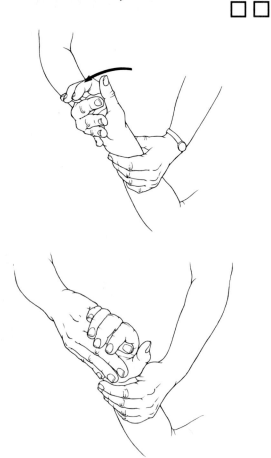

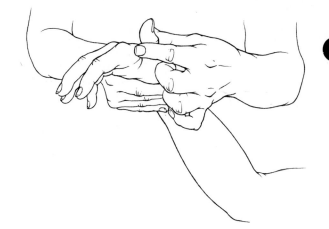

5. Drop the wrist down, pointing the person's thumb toward her toes. Then (*ulnar deviation*) bring the thumb up toward the person's nose (*radial deviation*). Repeat five times. ☐ ☐

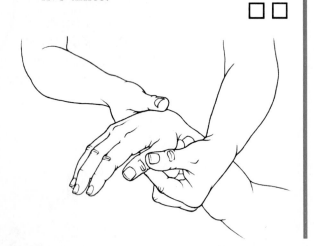

Task 4: Exercising the Fingers and Thumb

1. Hold the person's hand with one of your hands and support her wrist with your other hand. ☐ ☐

2. Flex the person's fingers to make a fist with the thumb tucked under the other fingers (*flexion*). Straighten the hand by extending the person's fingers, including the thumb, one at a time (*extension*). ☐ ☐

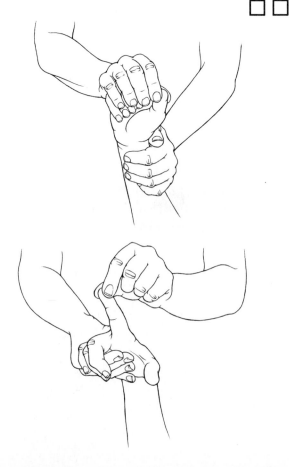

244

3. Hold the person's thumb and index finger together in one of your hands. With the other hand, spread her middle finger away from her index finger. Move it to the index finger and hold the middle finger, index finger, and thumb together. Move the ring finger away from the other three (thumb, index, and middle) then back to them. Hold all four. Do the same with the little finger. Then hold the little finger and ring finger together and move the middle finger away and back. Complete with index finger and thumb. (*abduction* and *adduction*). Repeat five times. ☐ ☐

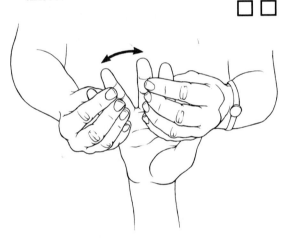

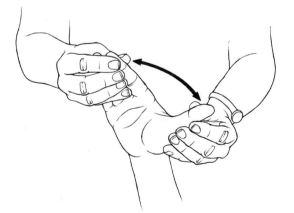

4. Bend the person's thumb in toward her palm and back next to the index finger (*abduction* and *adduction.*). ☐ ☐

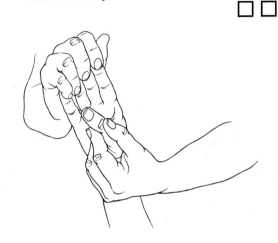

5. Bring the person's thumb to the tip of each finger (*thumb opposition*). Repeat five times. ☐ ☐

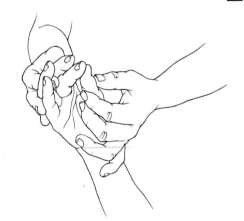

Task 5: Exercising the Hip and Knee

1. Put one hand under the person's knee and your other hand under her ankle. Provide this support throughout the following motions. ☐ ☐

2. Bend the person's knee and move it up toward her head to flex her knee and hip *(flexion)*. Repeat five times, alternating with extension. ☐ ☐

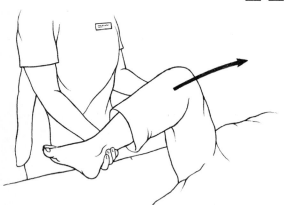

3. Straighten the person's knee to extend her knee and hip. Lower her leg to the bed *(extension)*. Repeat five times, alternating with flexion. ☐ ☐

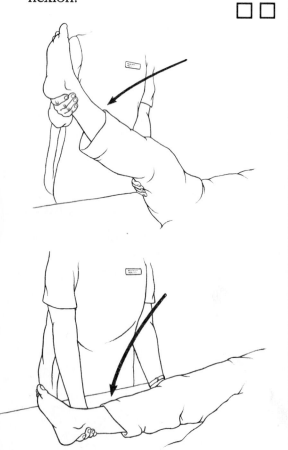

4. Move the person's leg out away from her body *(abduction)*. Repeat five times. ☐ ☐

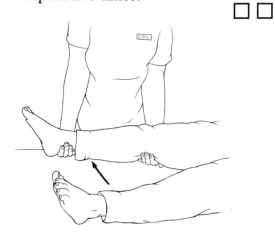

5. Move the person's leg back to the center toward his other leg *(adduction)*. Repeat five times. ☐ ☐

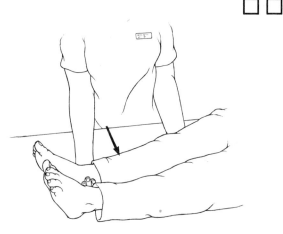

6. Turn the person's leg inward and then outward to rotate the hip *(rotation)*. Repeat five times. ☐ ☐

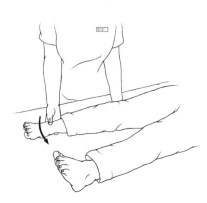

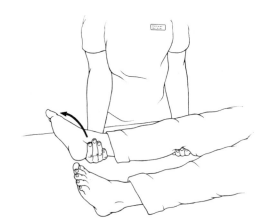

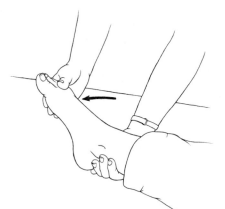

Task 6: Exercising the Ankle

1. Put one hand under the person's ankle and grasp her foot with your other hand. Provide this support throughout the following motions. ☐ ☐

2. Push the person's foot forward toward her head (*flexion*) and then downward (*extension*). Repeat five times. ☐ ☐

3. Turn the person's foot inward (*adduction*) and then outward (*abduction*). Repeat five times. ☐ ☐

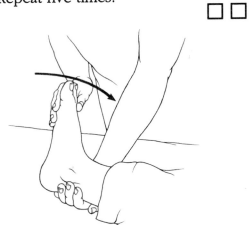

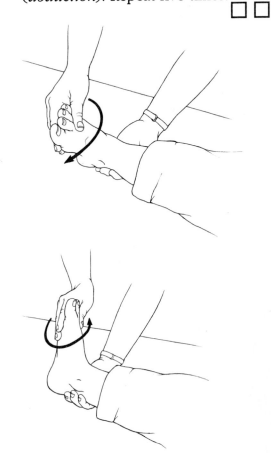

Task 7: Exercising the Toes

1. Put one hand under the person's foot and the other hand on the top of her foot over her toes. ☐ ☐

2. Curl her toes downward (*flexion*) and then straighten them (*extension*). ☐ ☐

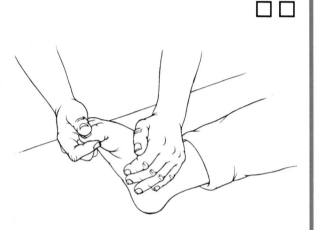

3. Holding two toes, spread each toe the same way you spread the fingers (*abduction* and *adduction*) in Task 4. ☐ ☐

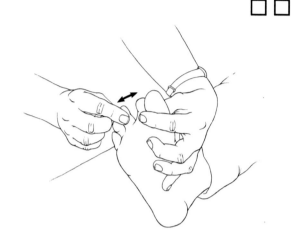

Note: Raise the side rail, if used, and move to the other side of the bed to repeat the sequence on the opposite side of the person's body.

Completion

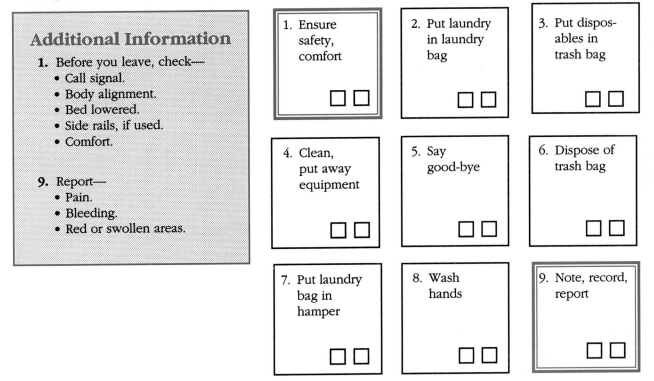

Additional Information

1. Before you leave, check—
   - Call signal.
   - Body alignment.
   - Bed lowered.
   - Side rails, if used.
   - Comfort.

9. Report—
   - Pain.
   - Bleeding.
   - Red or swollen areas.

1. Ensure safety, comfort ☐ ☐

2. Put laundry in laundry bag ☐ ☐

3. Put disposables in trash bag ☐ ☐

4. Clean, put away equipment ☐ ☐

5. Say good-bye ☐ ☐

6. Dispose of trash bag ☐ ☐

7. Put laundry bag in hamper ☐ ☐

8. Wash hands ☐ ☐

9. Note, record, report ☐ ☐

_____
Student   Date

_____
Instructor   Date

Skill 54: Helping a Person Walk

Precautions

- When a person is using a walker or cane, always be sure the rubber tips are in good shape.
- Always be sure to check how the person was taught to use the device to help him walk.
- Never use a safety belt if a person has—
- A recent colostomy or ileostomy.
- Severe heart problems.
- Had recent abdominal, chest, or back surgery.
- Severe respiratory problems.
- A fear of safety belts.
- When a person has an IV or catheter, make sure this equipment is cared for properly so that treatment is not disrupted and the person is not harmed. An IV always should be above the catheter entry site. A urinary catheter bag and tubing always should be below the bladder.

Preparation

1. Gather supplies
   - Walker, cane, or crutches, if needed. ☐ ☐

Additional Information

8. The person should wear sturdy, well-fitting shoes or slippers with nonskid soles.

---

2. Focus ☐ ☐

3. Knock and wait ☐ ☐

4. Introduce and identify ☐ ☐

5. Explain ☐ ☐

6. Place supplies ☐ ☐

7. Wash hands ☐ ☐

8. Gather and prepare ☐ ☐

9. Adjust bed ☐ ☐

10. Provide privacy ☐ ☐

Notes:

250

Procedure

Four different ways you can help with ambulation are assisting a person to walk:

1. With a walker.

2. With a cane.

3. With crutches.

4. Without a device.

Option 1: Assisting a Person to Walk with a Walker

1. Put a safety belt on the person as explained in Skill 18. Grip the safety belt as needed to support and assist the him. ☐ ☐

2. Put the walker directly in front of him. ☐ ☐

3. Help him to stand. ☐ ☐

4. Ask the person to put his hands on the walker's hand grips. The height of the walker should be at about the same height as his hip bone. ☐ ☐

5. Ask the person to flex his elbows slightly.

6. Remind him to stand erect. ☐ ☐

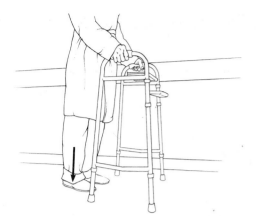

7. Have the person lift the walker and put it down about 6 inches forward and then step into it. Remind him to use the walker to support himself as he stands on his stronger leg and moves his weaker leg forward. He should use his arms to hold himself up if his legs are weak. ☐ ☐

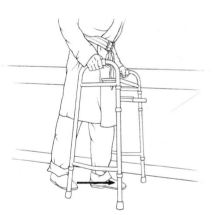

8. Remind the person to walk normally, looking ahead, while using the walker. ☐ ☐

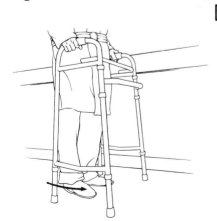

Option 2: Assisting a Person to Walk with a Cane

1. Put the safety belt on the person.

2. Help him to stand.

3. Put the cane near the person's stronger hand. Ask him to put his hand on the cane handle. Be certain that when the cane is at his side, the top of it is even with his hip bone and the bottom is 6 inches from his foot. ☐ ☐

4. Ask the person to flex his elbow slightly. ☐ ☐

5. Remind him to stand erect. ☐ ☐

6. Have the person use the cane to support himself as he stands on his stronger side and moves his weaker leg forward. ☐ ☐

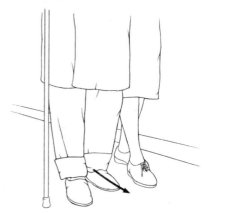

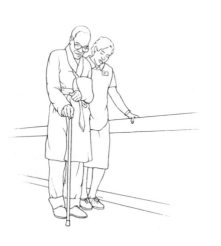

7. Walk on the weaker side of the person to assist him as necessary. ☐ ☐

8. Remind him to walk normally, looking ahead, while using the cane. ☐ ☐

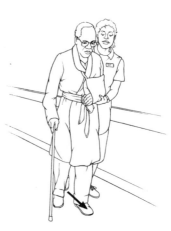

Option 3: Assisting a Person to Walk with Crutches

1. Put a safety belt on the person. ☐ ☐

2. Help him to stand. ☐ ☐

3. Give him the crutches. □ □

4. Help him place each crutch on either side, underneath his underarms. The nurse or physical therapist should adjust the crutches to the proper height for the person. □ □

5. Tell the person to extend his arms down along the crutches, putting his hands on the handgrips. □ □

6. Tell him to flex his elbows slightly. □ □

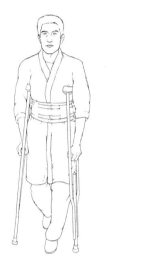

7. Remind him to stand erect. □ □

8. While the person is moving, he should support himself with his hands and by gripping the crutch between his chest and inside of his upper arm. □ □

Note: Remind the person not to lean on a crutch with his underarm because this can cause permanent injury to nerves in the area.

Stand behind the person and hold onto the safety belt.

9. Instruct him to move forward. □ □

Note: There are several different ways to walk with crutches. The method a person uses is determined by the amount of weight the person can bear on each foot and how strong his upper body is will determine the method he should use.

If the person can bear weight on both feet, have him follow these steps:
- Move the right crutch forward
- Move his left foot forward

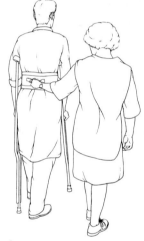

- Move the left crutch forward
- Move his right foot forward

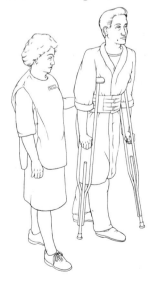

- Repeat these steps

The person also may move the right crutch and his left foot forward at the same time or the left crutch and his right foot forward at the same time.

If the person can bear weight on only one foot, have her:
- Move both crutches forward along with the weaker extremity.

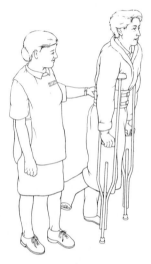

- Move her strong leg up to the crutches. (If her upper body is strong, the person may be able to swing her body through the crutches and have her good leg land past the crutches.)
- Repeat these steps.

10. Help the person practice the sequence with the left crutch and right foot, then the right crutch and left foot. ☐ ☐

11. Remind the person to look ahead while using the crutches. ☐ ☐

Option 4: Assisting a Person to Walk Without a Device

1. Put a safety belt on the person. ☐ ☐

2. Help him to stand. ☐ ☐

3. Stand at his side with your arm under his arm, holding his wrist. ☐ ☐

Note: If the person is weaker on one side than the other, stand on the weaker side so that you can support his ambulation. This may not be necessary at all times.

4. Hold the safety belt with an underhand grip or hold onto the back handles. Walk on the person's weaker side and a little behind the person. Discuss the options with your supervising nurse. ☐ ☐

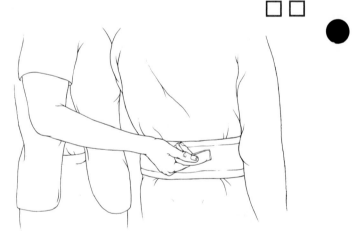

Note: You and the person should start on the same foot.

5. Remind the person to walk normally, looking ahead. ☐ ☐

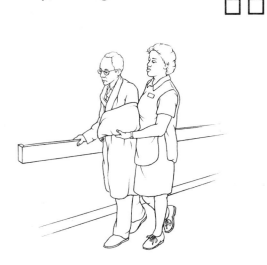

Note: People with poor balance will feel safer if they can watch the floor.

6. Gradually increase the distance the person walks to help build her confidence. ☐ ☐

Note: If the person in your care should fall:

- If possible, catch her. To maintain proper body mechanics, keep your feet apart, back straight, and knees slightly bent.

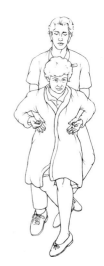

- Put your arms around her waist or underarms, keep her close to your body, bend your knees, and lower her slowly to the floor by sliding her down your leg.

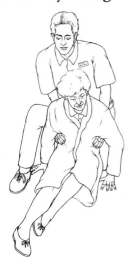

- Call for help.
- Help make the person comfortable by reassuring her and staying with her. Do not move her until she has been checked by a nurse and until you receive instructions to move her.

Review the section on first aid for falls Chapter 6, Keeping People Safe, in the textbook.

Completion

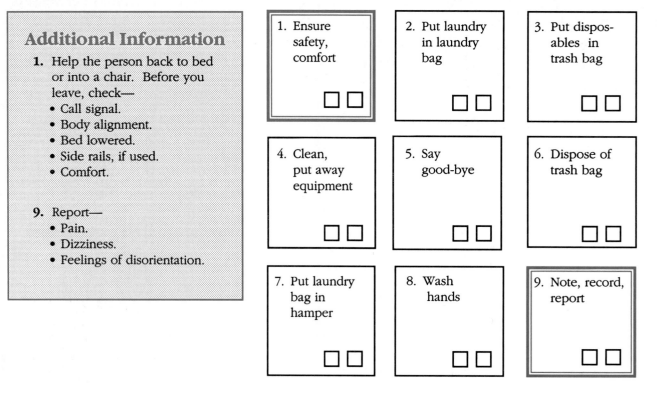

1. Ensure safety, comfort ☐ ☐

2. Put laundry in laundry bag ☐ ☐

3. Put disposables in trash bag ☐ ☐

4. Clean, put away equipment ☐ ☐

5. Say good-bye ☐ ☐

6. Dispose of trash bag ☐ ☐

7. Put laundry bag in hamper ☐ ☐

8. Wash hands ☐ ☐

9. Note, record, report ☐ ☐

_____

Student   Date

_____

Instructor   Date

256

Skill 55: Applying Elastic Stockings

Precautions

- Apply elastic stockings when a person has been lying down for at least 15 minutes. The best time to apply elastic stockings is before the person gets up in the morning. If the person has been standing, have him sit in a chair with his legs elevated for 15 minutes before applying the stockings.
- Check the person's toes for circulation every hour. Look for coldness or a bluish color.
- Ask the person if he has numbness or tingling in his feet. Remove the stockings and report to your supervising nurse if these symptoms occur.

Preparation

1. Gather supplies
   - Elastic stockings
   - Powder (optional)

   ☐ ☐

Additional Information

1. Elastic stockings come in various sizes. Check with your supervising nurse to be sure you have the correct size for the person.

2. Focus

   ☐ ☐

3. Knock and wait

   ☐ ☐

4. Introduce and identify

   ☐ ☐

5. Explain

   ☐ ☐

6. Place supplies

   ☐ ☐

7. Wash hands

   ☐ ☐

8. Gather and prepare

   ☐ ☐

9. Adjust bed

   ☐ ☐

10. Provide privacy

   ☐ ☐

Notes:

Procedure

1. Make sure the person is in a flat, supine position, if he can tolerate it. ☐ ☐

2. Lower the side rail, if used, on the side of the bed where you will be working. ☐ ☐

3. Pull the top sheet out from the bottom of the mattress and fold it back toward the person, exposing only his legs. ☐ ☐

4. Apply a small amount of powder to the person's lower legs and feet (optional).

Why? This will make it easier for the stockings to slide on.

5. Take one stocking and turn it inside out down to the heel. Put the stocking on the person's leg that is closest to you. Slide the stocking over the person's toes, foot, and heel. Position the opening across the toes. ☐ ☐

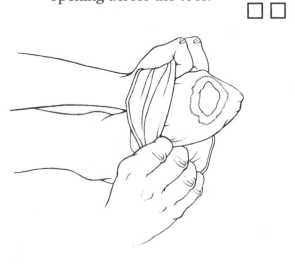

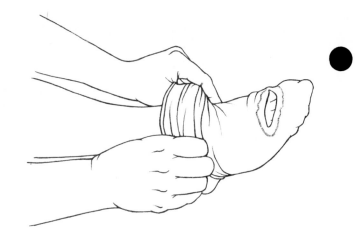

6. Slide the rest of the stocking up the leg smoothly. There should be no wrinkles in the stocking. ☐ ☐

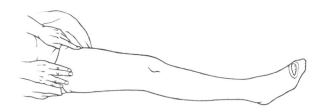

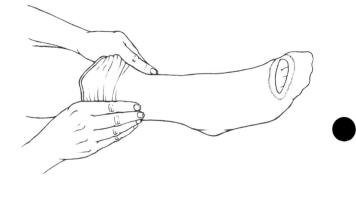

Why? Wrinkles can interfere with circulation.

258

7. Check the stocking to be sure it is not too tight across the person's toes.

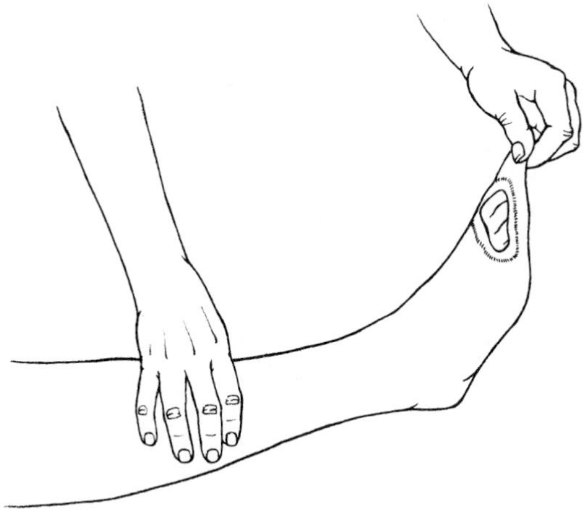

☐ ☐

8. Raise the side rail, if used. Go to the other side of the bed and lower the side rail.

☐ ☐

9. Repeat steps 5 through 8 to apply the stocking to the other leg.

☐ ☐

10. Replace the top sheet and raise the side rail, if used.

☐ ☐

Completion

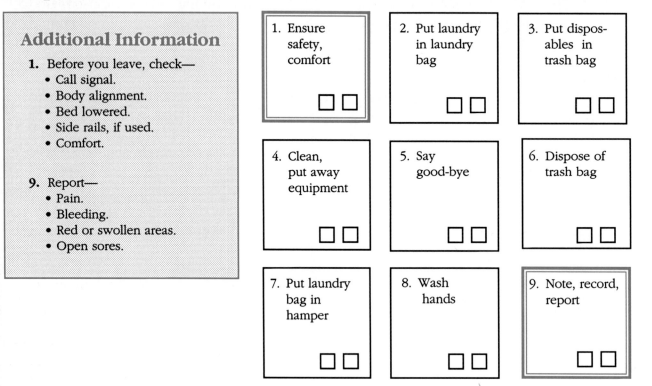

1. Ensure safety, comfort ☐ ☐

2. Put laundry in laundry bag ☐ ☐

3. Put disposables in trash bag ☐ ☐

4. Clean, put away equipment ☐ ☐

5. Say good-bye ☐ ☐

6. Dispose of trash bag ☐ ☐

7. Put laundry bag in hamper ☐ ☐

8. Wash hands ☐ ☐

9. Note, record, report ☐ ☐

_____   _____
Student   Date

_____   _____
Instructor   Date

Skill 56: Transferring a Person From Bed To Stretcher and Stretcher to Bed

Precautions

- Arrange for three co-workers to help you.
- Always lock the brakes on the bed and on the stretcher.
- Use the safety straps and side rails on the stretcher to secure the person as you are transporting him.
- Use proper body mechanics when transferring someone from the bed to the stretcher and from the stretcher to the bed.

Preparation

1. Gather supplies
   - Two disposable bed protectors
   - Top sheet
   - Bath blanket
   - Stretcher
   - Plastic trash bag
   - Laundry bag (or plastic bag for wet or soiled laundry)
   ☐ ☐

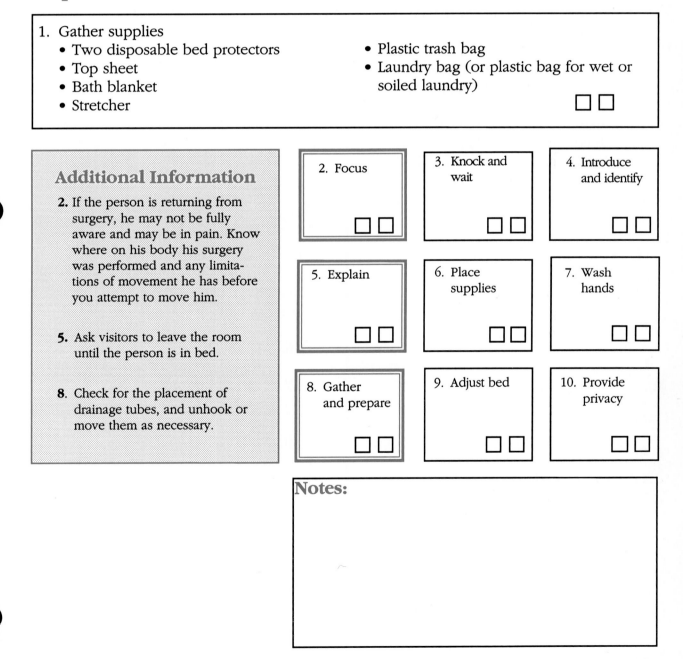

Additional Information

2. If the person is returning from surgery, he may not be fully aware and may be in pain. Know where on his body his surgery was performed and any limitations of movement he has before you attempt to move him.

5. Ask visitors to leave the room until the person is in bed.

8. Check for the placement of drainage tubes, and unhook or move them as necessary.

2. Focus ☐ ☐

3. Knock and wait ☐ ☐

4. Introduce and identify ☐ ☐

5. Explain ☐ ☐

6. Place supplies ☐ ☐

7. Wash hands ☐ ☐

8. Gather and prepare ☐ ☐

9. Adjust bed ☐ ☐

10. Provide privacy ☐ ☐

Notes:

Procedure:

Task 1: From Bed to Stretcher

1. You and a co-worker stand on one side of the bed. The other two nurse assistants stand on the other side of the bed. Lock the brakes on the bed. □ □

2. Position the stretcher close to the side of the bed to which the person will be moved. Leave enough space to stand between it and the bed. □ □

3. Lower the side rails. Cover the person with a bath blanket or sheet by placing it over the top bed linens. Ask the person to hold onto the blanket or sheet while you fold the top linens down to the foot of the bed. □ □

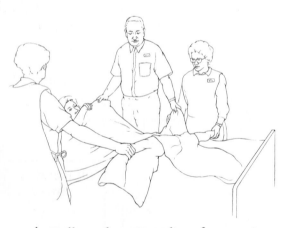

4. Follow the procedure for moving a person toward you to the side of the bed (see Skill 13). Leave the drawsheet untucked on top of the mattress. Stand close to the bed to keep the person from falling. □ □

Note: The head of the bed should still be in a flat position.

5. Have two of your co-workers on the opposite side of the bed hold the person's far arm and leg to protect her from falling while you and another co-worker position the stretcher at the side of the bed. □ □

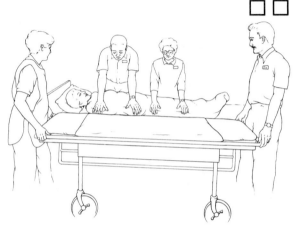

Note: Be sure the stretcher is flush against the bed. Leave no space between the bed and the stretcher. Make sure the drawsheet is on top of the mattress and not between the stretcher and the bed.

6. Lock the brakes on the stretcher. □ □

7. Have all nurse assistants roll the drawsheet toward the person. □ □

8. Ask the two nurse assistants on the side of the bed away from the stretcher to kneel on the empty half of the bed. □ □

Note: Each nurse assistant should place a disposable bed protector for infection control on the empty half of the bed.

9. With the help of all nurse assistants and at the count of three, lift the drawsheet with the palms of your hands facing up, and move the person onto the stretcher.

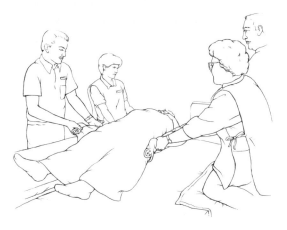

Make sure the person is centered on the stretcher and tighten the drawsheet. On the side of the stretcher farther from the bed, raise the side rail. One nurse assistant on the stretcher side should remain with the person for safety while another nurse assistant should move to the other side of the stretcher to unlock the brakes and move the stretcher away from the side of the bed. ☐ ☐

10. Fasten the safety belts and raise the other side rail. Make sure that the person is covered. Check her for proper body alignment and make sure she is comfortable. Check for the placement of drainage tubes. ☐ ☐

11. With a co-worker, transport the person to her destination. One of you walks at the head of the stretcher, while the other walks at the foot. ☐ ☐

Task 2: From Stretcher to Bed

1. You and a co-worker stand on one side of the bed. The other two nurse assistants stand on the other side of the bed. Lock the brakes on the bed. ☐ ☐

2. Adjust the height of the bed so that it is at the height of the stretcher. ☐ ☐

3. Lower the side rail on the side of the *bed* where you will be placing the stretcher. ☐ ☐

4. Lower the side rail on the side of the *stretcher* that you will be placing against the bed. Loosen the drawsheet on that side and place it on top of the stretcher mattress. ☐ ☐

5. Place the stretcher against the side of the bed and lock the brakes. ☐ ☐

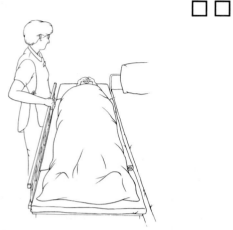

6. Lower the other side rail of the stretcher and loosen the draw sheet on that side. ☐ ☐

Note: Keep the person covered with a sheet.

7. Ask the two nurse assistants standing on the other side of the bed to lower the side rail, place disposable bed protectors on the bed, and then kneel on the bed. ☐ ☐

8. Have all nurse assistants roll the drawsheet toward the person. At the count of three, lift the drawsheet with the palms of your hands facing up, and move the person to the side of the bed. The two nurse assistants kneeling on the bed will return to a standing position. They will hold the person in place, while the two other nurse assistants unlock and remove the stretcher, and then return to the bedside. ☐ ☐

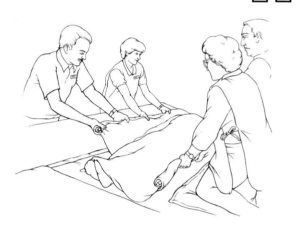

9. Position the person in the middle of the bed and either remove the extra drawsheet or tighten and smooth it. ☐ ☐

10. Raise the side rails, if used. ☐ ☐

Completion

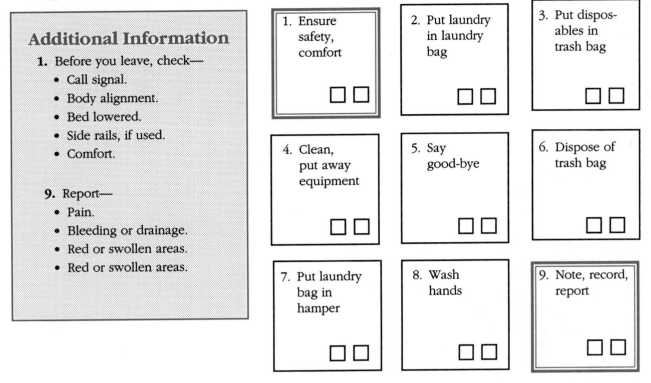

1. Ensure safety, comfort ☐ ☐

2. Put laundry in laundry bag ☐ ☐

3. Put disposables in trash bag ☐ ☐

4. Clean, put away equipment ☐ ☐

5. Say good-bye ☐ ☐

6. Dispose of trash bag ☐ ☐

7. Put laundry bag in hamper ☐ ☐

8. Wash hands ☐ ☐

9. Note, record, report ☐ ☐

_____

Student   Date

_____

Instructor   Date

Skill 57: Making a Postop or Surgical Bed

Preparation

1. Gather supplies
   - Pillow case
   - Top sheet
   - Drawsheet
   - Two bath blankets
   - Bottom sheet
   - Laundry bag
   - IV pole
   ☐ ☐

Additional Information

8. Gather the person's own—
   - Emesis basin (small, kidney-shaped basin designed to catch emesis, which is the vomited content of the stomach; also used to catch other fluids from the mouth).
   - Tissues.

2. Focus
   ☐ ☐

3. Knock and wait
   ☐ ☐

4. Introduce and identify
   ☐ ☐

5. Explain
   ☐ ☐

6. Place supplies
   ☐ ☐

7. Wash hands
   ☐ ☐

8. Gather and prepare
   ☐ ☐

9. Adjust bed
   ☐ ☐

10. Provide privacy
    ☐ ☐

Notes:

Procedure

1. Remove dirty linens from bed and make the bottom of the bed as you would for an unoccupied bed (see Skill 35). Place one bath blanket on top of the drawsheet and tuck it in. ☐ ☐

Why? People frequently feel cold after anesthesia. A blanket adds warmth.

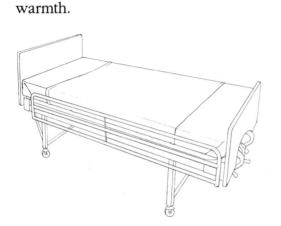

2. Place the second bath blanket folded lengthwise on the bed about 12 inches from the top of the mattress with the fold in the center of the mattress. Unfold the blanket so that it is hangs evenly on both sides of the bed. ☐ ☐

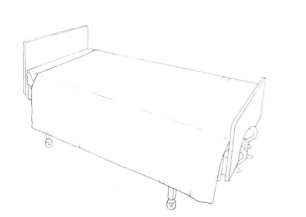

3. Place the top sheet, blanket, and spread in the usual manner, but do not tuck in at the bottom of the mattress. ☐ ☐

4. Fold back the top and bottom of the linens one-fourth of the way. ☐ ☐

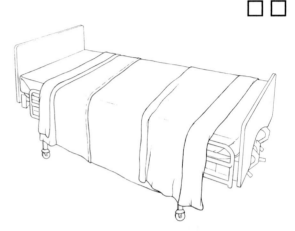

5. Fanfold the top linens lengthwise to the side of the bed farthest from the door or fold to the bottom of the bed. ☐ ☐

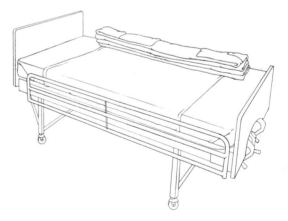

6. Cover the pillow with a clean pillowcase and place it up against the headboard. ☐ ☐

7. Place the IV pole near the head of the bed.

□ □

8. Place the emesis basin and tissues on the bedside table.

□ □

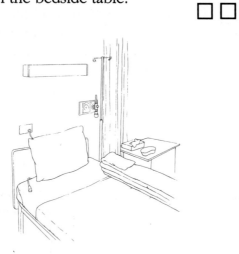

9. Make room for the stretcher to be moved against the bed. Leave the bed in its highest position.

□ □

Completion

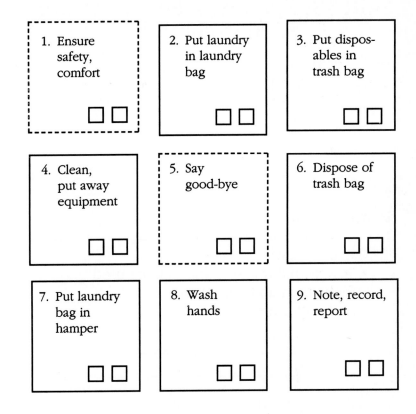

1. Ensure safety, comfort	2. Put laundry in laundry bag	3. Put disposables in trash bag
☐ ☐	☐ ☐	☐ ☐
4. Clean, put away equipment	5. Say good-bye	6. Dispose of trash bag
☐ ☐	☐ ☐	☐ ☐
7. Put laundry bag in hamper	8. Wash hands	9. Note, record, report
☐ ☐	☐ ☐	☐ ☐

_____

Student   Date

_____

Instructor   Date

Skill 58: Turning a Person Using a Log-Rolling Technique

Precautions

- Arrange for help from another co-worker.

Preparation

1. Gather supplies • Towels, pillows, or blankets to be used for support and positioning • Bed protectors   ☐ ☐

Additional Information

2. Remember that the person may be fearful or in pain.

9. The bed should be at waist level.

2. Focus ☐ ☐	3. Knock and wait ☐ ☐	4. Introduce and identify ☐ ☐
5. Explain ☐ ☐	6. Place supplies ☐ ☐	7. Wash hands ☐ ☐
8. Gather and prepare ☐ ☐	9. Adjust bed ☐ ☐	10. Provide privacy ☐ ☐

Notes:

Procedure

1. Ask your co-worker to stand on same side of the bed with you. Lower the side rail, if used. ☐ ☐

2. Place your hands under the person's head and shoulders. ☐ ☐

3. Ask your co-worker to place his or her hands under the person's hips and legs. ☐ ☐

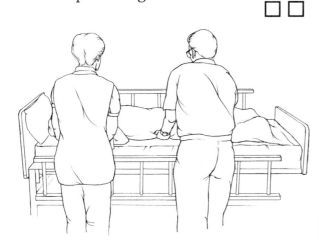

4. Stand with one foot slightly behind the other and on the count of three rock backwards, transferring your weight to the back foot and moving the person toward the side of the bed as a unit. ☐ ☐

5. Raise the side rail, if used. ☐ ☐

6. Lower the bed so that you can put one knee on the bed and still place your other foot flat on the floor. ☐ ☐

7. With your co-workers, go to the opposite side of the bed. ☐ ☐

8. Lower the side rail, if used. Place a pillow between the person's knees. Cross the person's arms over her chest. ☐ ☐

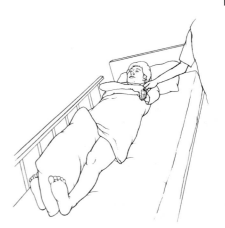

Along with your co-worker, place a bed protector on the bed and place one knee on top of the bed protector.

9. Place your hands on the person's far shoulder and hips. ☐ ☐

10. Ask your co-worker to place his or her hands on the person's far thigh and lower leg. ☐ ☐

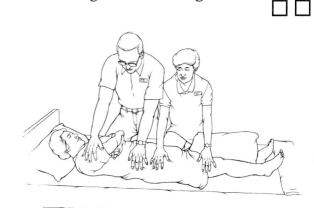

11. On the count of three, turn the person on her side keeping her head, back, and legs in a straight line. ☐ ☐

12. Check to see that the pillow between the person's legs is still in place. ☐ ☐

13. Position pillows behind the person's spine to maintain the position. Support her top arm with pillows or folded blankets. If allowed, place a small pillow or folded blanket under her head. ☐ ☐

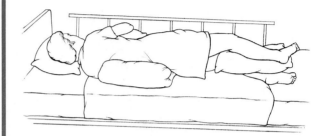

Completion

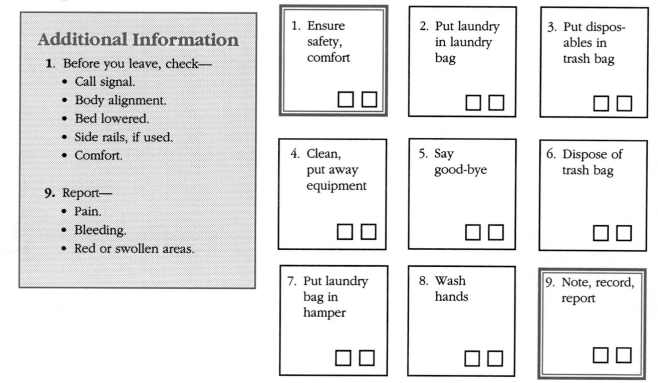

Additional Information

1. Before you leave, check—
- Call signal.
- Body alignment.
- Bed lowered.
- Side rails, if used.
- Comfort.

9. Report—
- Pain.
- Bleeding.
- Red or swollen areas.

1. Ensure safety, comfort ☐ ☐

2. Put laundry in laundry bag ☐ ☐

3. Put disposables in trash bag ☐ ☐

4. Clean, put away equipment ☐ ☐

5. Say good-bye ☐ ☐

6. Dispose of trash bag ☐ ☐

7. Put laundry bag in hamper ☐ ☐

8. Wash hands ☐ ☐

9. Note, record, report ☐ ☐

_____

Student   Date

_____

Instructor   Date

Skill 59: Cleaning Around Tubes and Catheters

Precautions

- Soap may irritate the skin.
- Do not pull on tubes or catheters, because they might become dislodged.

Preparation

1. Gather supplies
   - Washcloth
   - Lubricant, if needed
   - Disposable gloves
   - Cotton-tip applicator
   - Antibacterial cream or lotion, if directed
   - Mild soap, if needed
   - Towel
   - Plastic trash bag ☐ ☐

Additional Information

2. You must clean areas surrounding nasogastric tubes, such as oxygen cannulas, catheters, and similar tubes. Because these tubes often are inserted through the person's nostril, her nose needs internal and external care.

8. Basin of warm water.

2. Focus ☐ ☐	3. Knock and wait ☐ ☐	4. Introduce and identify ☐ ☐
5. Explain ☐ ☐	6. Place supplies ☐ ☐	7. Wash hands ☐ ☐
8. Gather and prepare ☐ ☐	9. Adjust bed ☐ ☐	10. Provide privacy ☐ ☐

Notes:

Procedure

1. Lower the side rail, if used. ☐ ☐

2. Put on disposable gloves. ☐ ☐

3. Drape a towel over the person's chest ☐ ☐

4. Use warm water and a washcloth to gently remove any mucus or secretions that collect around the tube. ☐ ☐

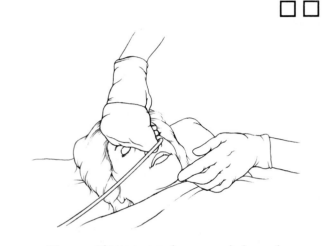

Note: Always wash around the tube without putting pressure on it. Mild soap may be used to clean the area, but it may irritate the skin.

5. Rinse the skin thoroughly and dry with the towel. Your supervising nurse may instruct you to use a lubricant if the person's nose is irritated. An antibacterial cream or lotion also may be applied, if directed. ☐ ☐

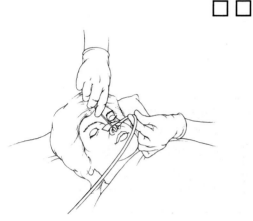

6. Raise the side rail, if used. ☐ ☐

7. Take off the disposable gloves and throw them in the plastic trash bag. ☐ ☐

Completion

Additional Information

1. Before you leave, check—
- Call signal.
- Body alignment.
- Bed lowered.
- Side rails, if used.
- Comfort.

9. Report—
- Pain.
- Bleeding or drainage.
- Red or swollen areas.
- Skin discoloration.

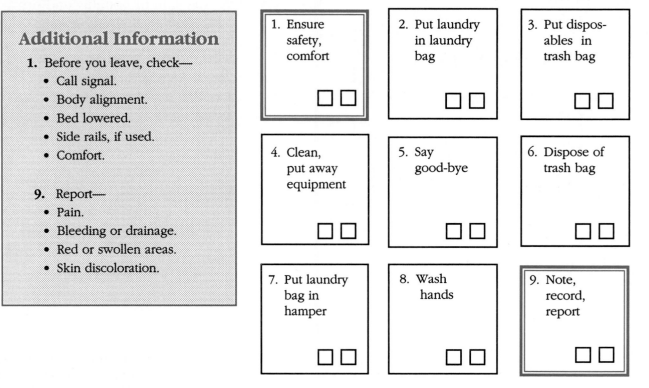

1. Ensure safety, comfort ☐ ☐

2. Put laundry in laundry bag ☐ ☐

3. Put disposables in trash bag ☐ ☐

4. Clean, put away equipment ☐ ☐

5. Say good-bye ☐ ☐

6. Dispose of trash bag ☐ ☐

7. Put laundry bag in hamper ☐ ☐

8. Wash hands ☐ ☐

9. Note, record, report ☐ ☐

_____

Student   Date

_____

Instructor   Date

Skill 60: Sterilizing Glass Baby Bottles

Precautions

- You may boil glass baby bottles, but check with the client before boiling plastic bottles.

Preparation

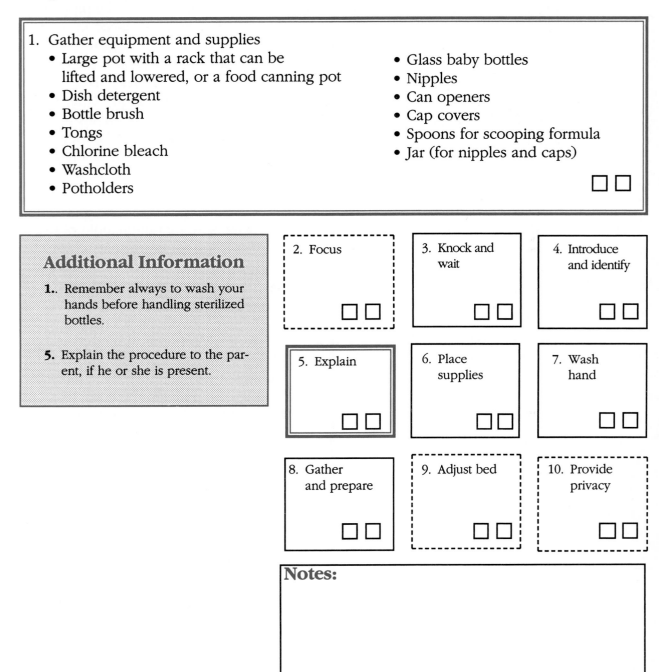

1. Gather equipment and supplies
   - Large pot with a rack that can be lifted and lowered, or a food canning pot
   - Dish detergent
   - Bottle brush
   - Tongs
   - Chlorine bleach
   - Washcloth
   - Potholders
   - Glass baby bottles
   - Nipples
   - Can openers
   - Cap covers
   - Spoons for scooping formula
   - Jar (for nipples and caps)

Additional Information

1.. Remember always to wash your hands before handling sterilized bottles.

5. Explain the procedure to the parent, if he or she is present.

2. Focus

3. Knock and wait

4. Introduce and identify

5. Explain

6. Place supplies

7. Wash hand

8. Gather and prepare

9. Adjust bed

10. Provide privacy

Notes:

Procedure

1. Using hot soapy water and a bottle brush, scrub the bottles, nipples, caps, and tongs. For bottles with disposable plastic liners, wash all items and then sterilize just the nipples, rings and disks, and nipple covers. ☐ ☐

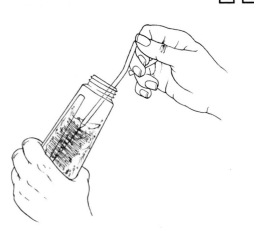

2. Rinse all items under hot, running water. Squeeze water through the holes in the nipples to make sure they are free of formula or milk particles. ☐ ☐

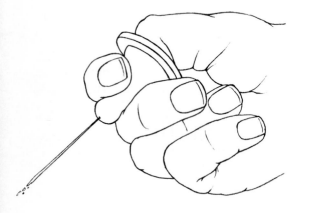

3. Use a large pot that has a rack that can be lifted and lowered like a food canning pot. Place it on the stove. Place the bottles upside down on the rack, along with the nipples, can openers, cap covers, spoons for scooping formula, and tongs. The nipples and caps may be placed in open jars to keep them together. Lower the rack into the pot. If the pot does not have a rack, place a clean dish towel in the bottom of the pot and put the bottles in the pot upside down. Add enough water to measure 3 inches from the bottom of the pot. ☐ ☐

4. Cover the pot with a lid and make sure that the handle of the pot is turned inward, for safety. ☐ ☐

5. Turn on the stove and bring the water to a boil. Let it boil for 20 minutes to kill most harmful germs. Do not lift the lid. ☐ ☐

6. At the end of 20 minutes, turn off the heat and allow the pot to cool for a few minutes before removing it from the burner. ☐ ☐

7. While the bottles and other equipment are sterilizing, thoroughly clean a counter area by sanitizing it with chlorine bleach, wiping it with clear water, and allowing it to dry. You also may use a thoroughly cleaned and sanitized flat cooling rack placed on a sanitized counter top to drain bottles and equipment. ☐ ☐

8. Using pot holders, lift the rack and allow it to drain on the sanitized area. If your pot does not have a rack, use a utensil to lift the tongs by the handle from the pot. Allow the tong handles to cool enough to use. Use the tongs to remove the bottles and other items. Place them inverted on the sanitized area to drain and cool. ☐ ☐

9. Before touching the bottles and equipment again, wash your hands. Assemble nipples and cap bottles and store them in a convenient location at room temperature. Do not touch the nipple tips or the inside of the bottles. ☐ ☐

10. If you need to sterilize other items, ask your supervisor for directions. ☐ ☐

Completion

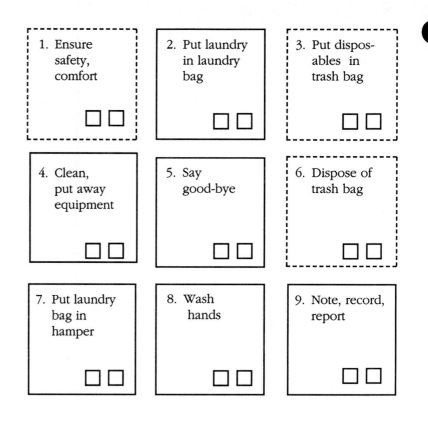

1. Ensure safety, comfort ☐ ☐	2. Put laundry in laundry bag ☐ ☐	3. Put disposables in trash bag ☐ ☐
4. Clean, put away equipment ☐ ☐	5. Say good-bye ☐ ☐	6. Dispose of trash bag ☐ ☐
7. Put laundry bag in hamper ☐ ☐	8. Wash hands ☐ ☐	9. Note, record, report ☐ ☐

_____

Student   Date

_____

Instructor   Date

Skill 61: Bathing a Newborn

Precautions

- Make sure the room is warm.
- Be sure to have everything within reach before starting the bath, because you cannot leave the baby after the bath has started.
- Wash the baby from the cleanest to the dirtiest part—face first, then torso, arms, legs, and bottom.
- Avoid getting the baby's umbilical cord wet.

Preparation

1. Gather supplies
   - Washcloth
   - Mild soap
   - Shampoo
   - Water warm to the touch in a bathtub, pan, or sink
   - Two towels
   - Clean clothing and diaper
   - Blanket
   - Petroleum jelly and cotton swab, if needed for circumcision care
   - Alcohol wipe or cotton balls and alcohol
   - Disposable gloves

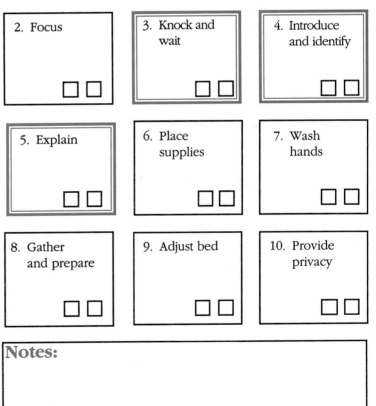

Additional Information

3. Wait for the baby's parent, if present, to reply.

4. Talk to the infant as you work. Introduce yourself to the parent, if one is present.

5. Explain your tasks to the parent, if one is present.

2. Focus

3. Knock and wait

4. Introduce and identify

5. Explain

6. Place supplies

7. Wash hands

8. Gather and prepare

9. Adjust bed

10. Provide privacy

Notes:

Procedure

1. Undress the baby, except for the diaper, and place the baby on a towel. □ □

2. Make sure the water temperature is correct, warm to the touch.

3. Make a mitt and wash the baby's face with a washcloth dipped in plain water. Gently wipe each closed eye from the inner to the outer corner with a different side of the mitt. Pat dry with the clean towel. □ □

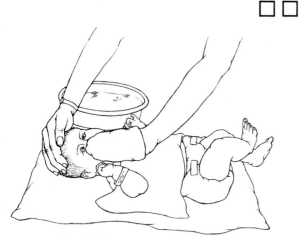

4. Clean the outside of the baby's ears and behind the ears with the washcloth and plain water. You don't need to clean the inside the baby's ears farther than you can reach with the washcloth. Avoid using cotton swabs because they can cause damage to the ears. □ □

5. Shampoo the baby's head by holding the baby in a football hold over the basin. Use the washcloth to wet the head. Apply a small amount of shampoo and wash it. Rinse by using the washcloth to squeeze water over the baby's head. Use the towel to dry it. □ □

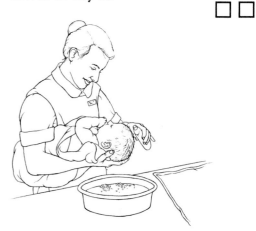

6. Lay the baby back down on the towel and remove the diaper. Using the mitted washcloth and soap, wash the baby's arms, chest, legs, back, genital area, and buttocks. Keep the cord area dry. Rinse and pat dry, especially between skin creases. □ □

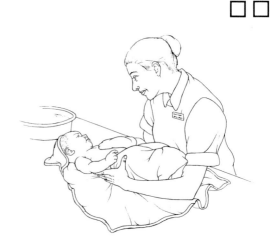

7. Put on disposable gloves. ☐ ☐

8. Provide care for the cord (and circumcision, if needed). ☐ ☐

9. Remove gloves and discard in the plastic trash bag. ☐ ☐

10. Put a clean diaper and clothes on the baby. ☐ ☐

Completion

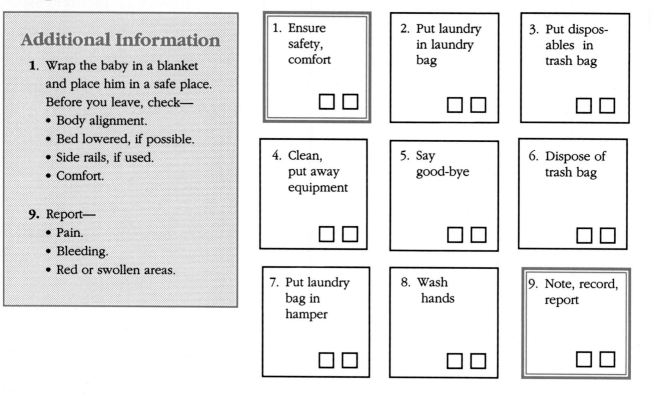

1. Ensure safety, comfort □ □

2. Put laundry in laundry bag □ □

3. Put disposables in trash bag □ □

4. Clean, put away equipment □ □

5. Say good-bye □ □

6. Dispose of trash bag □ □

7. Put laundry bag in hamper □ □

8. Wash hands □ □

9. Note, record, report □ □

_____
Student   Date

_____
Instructor   Date

Skill 62: Providing Postmortem Care

Precautions

- Put on disposable gloves for infection control.

Preparation

1. **Gather supplies.**
   - One or two pairs of disposable gloves
   - Disposable bed protector
   - One or two completed identification tags
   - Clean sheet
   - Washcloth
   - Soap
   - Shroud (optional)
   - Plastic trash bag
   - Laundry bag (or plastic bag for wet or soiled linens)

   ☐ ☐

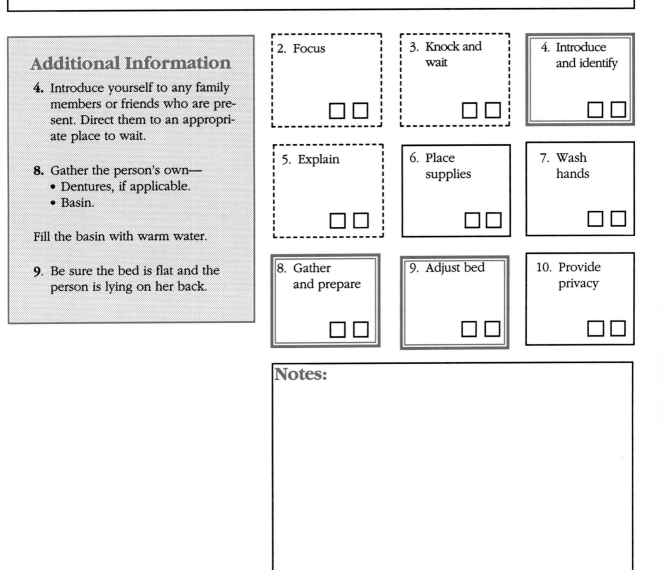

Additional Information

4. Introduce yourself to any family members or friends who are present. Direct them to an appropriate place to wait.

8. Gather the person's own—
   - Dentures, if applicable.
   - Basin.

   Fill the basin with warm water.

9. Be sure the bed is flat and the person is lying on her back.

2. Focus ☐ ☐

3. Knock and wait ☐ ☐

4. Introduce and identify ☐ ☐

5. Explain ☐ ☐

6. Place supplies ☐ ☐

7. Wash hands ☐ ☐

8. Gather and prepare ☐ ☐

9. Adjust bed ☐ ☐

10. Provide privacy ☐ ☐

Notes:

Procedure

1. Put on disposable gloves. ☐ ☐

2. When your supervising nurse has given you permission, remove any equipment, tubes, clothing, or jewelry from the person.

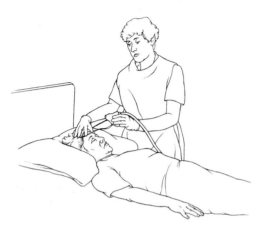

3. Replace the person's dentures if your supervising nurse tells you to.

Why? Replacing dentures keeps the person's face from losing its normal appearance.

4. Close the person's eyes and mouth. Close the eyelids by holding the lashes and gently pulling the lids over the eyes.

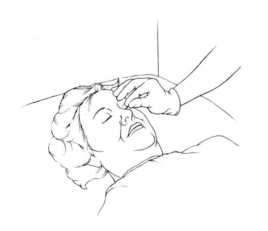

Why? Touching the eyelids themselves may give the eyes an unnatural appearance.

5. Clean the person's body. ☐ ☐

Why? Body fluids often ooze out of the body.

6. Put a disposable bed protector under the person's buttocks to absorb any fecal material. ☐ ☐

7. Cover the person with a clean sheet. ☐ ☐

Why? Covering the person maintains privacy and dignity.

8. Put an identification tag around the person's ankle. ☐ ☐

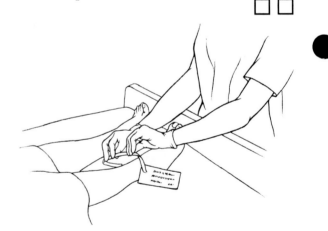

Why? This assists the morgue with identification.

9. If your employer permits it and the family wishes it, allow family members to view the person's body.

10. If it is your employer's policy, wrap the person's body in a shroud. To do this, place the body on the shroud and then either zip it together or fold the ends over and tape them to enclose the body. Follow these steps to fold a shroud:

- Fold the top down over the person's head.
- Fold the bottom up over her feet.

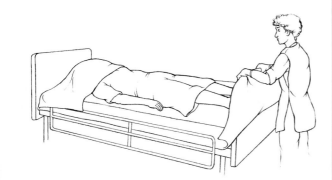

- Fold the sides over the person's body and tape the ends together.

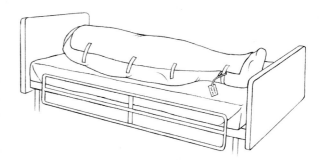

Attach an identification tag to the shroud.

Note: A shroud is a baglike garment used to hold a dead person's body.

11. Remove the disposable gloves and discard in the plastic trash bag.

☐ ☐

Completion

Additional Information

9. Collect all of the person's belongings. Check them against the valuables list. Put the belongings in a bag and label the bag for the person's family.

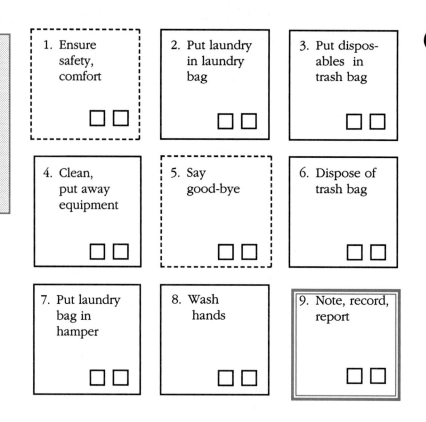

1. Ensure safety, comfort ☐ ☐

2. Put laundry in laundry bag ☐ ☐

3. Put disposables in trash bag ☐ ☐

4. Clean, put away equipment ☐ ☐

5. Say good-bye ☐ ☐

6. Dispose of trash bag ☐ ☐

7. Put laundry bag in hamper ☐ ☐

8. Wash hands ☐ ☐

9. Note, record, report ☐ ☐

_____
Student   Date

_____
Instructor   Date

Skill 63: Applying Compresses and Assisting with Soaks

Precautions

- High temperatures can burn skin. Immediately report any signs of burns, pain, redness, or blisters.
- Babies, young children, and elderly people are injured more easily by heat or cold, because their skin is more delicate.
- Be especially careful in applying heat to a person who is confused or who has poor sensation in the affected area.
- Prolonged or intense cold can damage skin and cause blisters, pain, or redness. Signs of cold damage may include pale, white, or bluish color of skin; pain; numbness; or tingling.

Preparation

1. Gather supplies
   - Two towels
   - Washcloth or gauze for compress
   - Disposable bed protector
   - Watch
   - Bath thermometer
   - Laundry bag (or plastic bag for wet or soiled linens)
   - Disposable gloves
   - Plastic trash bag

   ☐ ☐

Additional Information

8. Fill the washbasin with water. Ask your supervising nurse what the temperature of the water should be and what the proper length of time for applying the compress or soaking should be.

2. Focus

   ☐ ☐

3. Knock and wait

   ☐ ☐

4. Introduce and identify

   ☐ ☐

5. Explain

   ☐ ☐

6. Place supplies

   ☐ ☐

7. Wash hands

   ☐ ☐

8. Gather and prepare

   ☐ ☐

9. Adjust bed

   ☐ ☐

10. Provide privacy

   ☐ ☐

Notes:

Procedure

Applying a Warm or Cold Compress

1. Lower the side rail, if used, on the side of the bed where you will be working. ☐ ☐

2. Protect the bed linens with a disposable bed protector. Position a towel half-way under the affected area. ☐ ☐

3. Put on disposable gloves. ☐ ☐

4. Dip the washcloth or gauze into the washbasin of warm water. Wring out any excess moisture. ☐ ☐

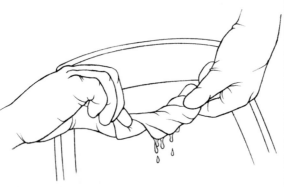

5. Gently place the compress on the affected area of the person's skin. ☐ ☐

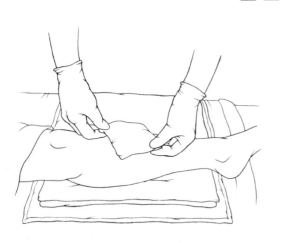

6. Place the other half of the towel over the compress and protect it with the disposable bed protector. ☐ ☐

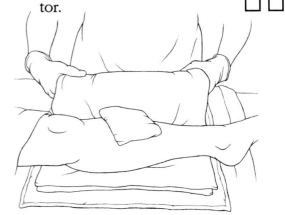

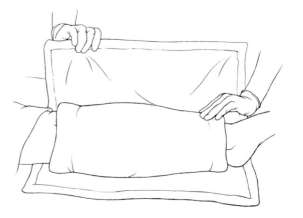

7. Use your watch to keep track of the amount of time the compress remains on the person's skin. ☐ ☐

8. Remove the compress and reapply it as needed. ☐ ☐

9. When the time is up, gently dry the affected area gently with the clean towel. ☐ ☐

10. Remove the disposable gloves and discard them in the plastic trash bag.

11. Raise the side rail, if used.

Assisting with a Warm Soak

1. Lower the side rail, if used, on the side of the bed where you will be working. ☐ ☐

2. Place the disposable bed protector on the bed or a clean surface. ☐ ☐

3. Place the washbasin on the bed protector and place the area to be treated in the water in the basin. ☐ ☐

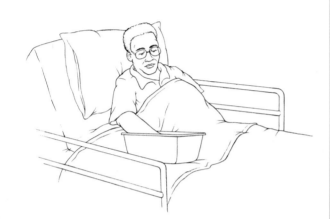

4. Use your watch to time the soak. ☐ ☐

5. When the time is up, gently dry the area with a clean towel. ☐ ☐

6. Remove the washbasin and disposable bed protector. Discard the bed protector in the plastic trash bag. ☐ ☐

7. Raise the side rail, if used. ☐ ☐

Completion

Additional Information

1. Before you leave, check—
- Call signal.
- Body alignment.
- Bed lowered.
- Side rails, if used..
- Comfort.

9. Record—
- Duration of application.
- Location of application.
- Time of application.
- Person's response to the application.

Report—
- Pain.
- Red or swollen areas.

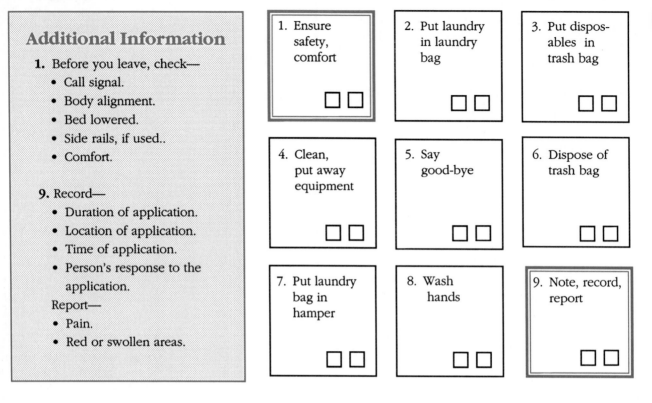

1. Ensure safety, comfort □ □

2. Put laundry in laundry bag □ □

3. Put disposables in trash bag □ □

4. Clean, put away equipment □ □

5. Say good-bye □ □

6. Dispose of trash bag □ □

7. Put laundry bag in hamper □ □

8. Wash hands □ □

9. Note, record, report □ □

_____

Student   Date

_____

Instructor   Date

Skill 64: Applying a Heat Lamp

Precautions

- Always follow the doctor's orders for heat lamp application.
- Never apply a heat lamp for more than 5 minutes, because heat lamps can cause burns quickly.
- Always stay with the person during the application so that you can monitor the heat applied to the skin.
- Check the skin often for the following signs of burning: redness, blistering, or pain.
- Keep linens away from the lamp to prevent them from catching fire.
- Caution the person not to move during the treatment.

Preparation

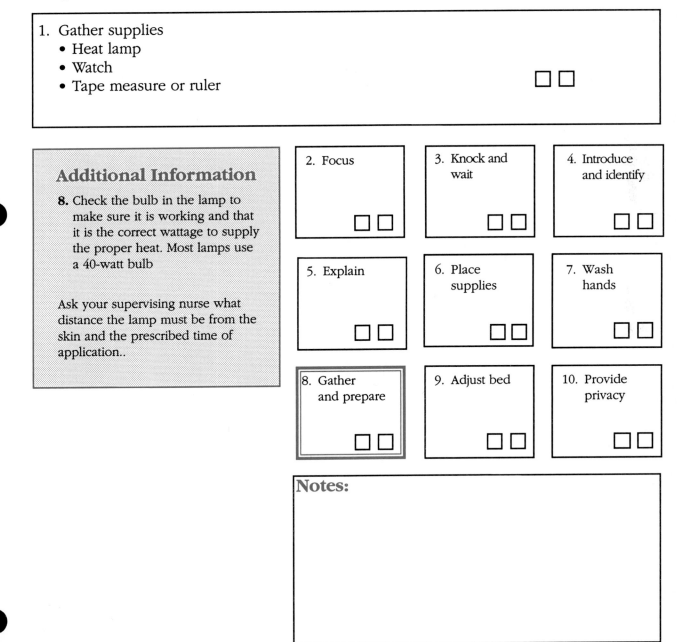

1. Gather supplies
   - Heat lamp
   - Watch
   - Tape measure or ruler

   ☐ ☐

Additional Information

8. Check the bulb in the lamp to make sure it is working and that it is the correct wattage to supply the proper heat. Most lamps use a 40-watt bulb

Ask your supervising nurse what distance the lamp must be from the skin and the prescribed time of application..

2. Focus ☐ ☐

3. Knock and wait ☐ ☐

4. Introduce and identify ☐ ☐

5. Explain ☐ ☐

6. Place supplies ☐ ☐

7. Wash hands ☐ ☐

8. Gather and prepare ☐ ☐

9. Adjust bed ☐ ☐

10. Provide privacy ☐ ☐

Notes:

Procedure

1. Lower the side rail, if used, on the side where you will be positioning the lamp. ☐ ☐

2. Fold back the bed linens or the bath blanket to expose the person's affected skin area. ☐ ☐

3. Position the heat lamp according to the doctor's orders by measuring the lamp's distance from the skin with a ruler or tape measure. ☐ ☐

4. Plug in the lamp. ☐ ☐

5. Time the application for the prescribed time and stay with the person during this time. ☐ ☐

Note: During the application, check the person's skin for redness and blistering. Ask the person if he feels any pain. If the person reports pain or burning, stop the treatment and immediately report this information to your supervising nurse.

6. Turn off the lamp when the time is up, and move it away from the person. ☐ ☐

7. Raise the side rail, if used. ☐ ☐

Completion

Additional Information

1. Before you leave, check—
   - Call signal.
   - Body alignment.
   - Bed lowered.
   - Side rails, if used.
   - Comfort.
9. Record—
   - Duration of application.
   - Location of application.
   - Time of application.
   - Person's response to application.

   Report—
   - Pain.
   - Red or swollen areas.

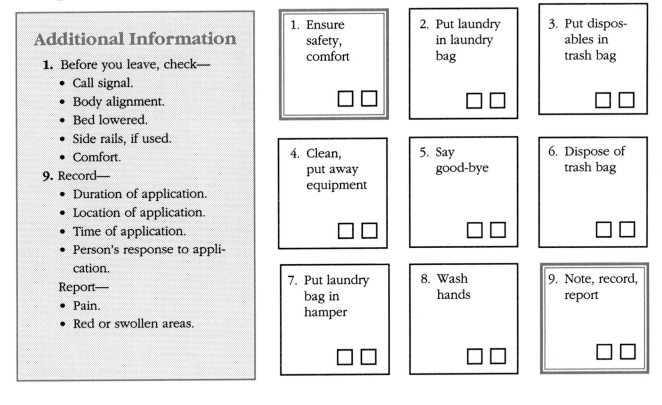

1. Ensure safety, comfort ☐ ☐

2. Put laundry in laundry bag ☐ ☐

3. Put disposables in trash bag ☐ ☐

4. Clean, put away equipment ☐ ☐

5. Say good-bye ☐ ☐

6. Dispose of trash bag ☐ ☐

7. Put laundry bag in hamper ☐ ☐

8. Wash hands ☐ ☐

9. Note, record, report ☐ ☐

_____

Student   Date

_____

Instructor   Date

Skill 65: Applying a Heating Pad

Precautions

- Never use pins to secure an electric heating pad.
- Make sure the temperature setting is correct. High temperatures can cause a person's skin to burn.
- Keep the heating pad from getting wet.
- Make sure the person's skin is clean and dry before applying the heating pad.
- Do not allow the person to lie on top of a heating pad, because lying on it increases the likelihood of burns.
- If the heating pad does not have a cloth surface or flannel cover, place a towel around it before placing it on the person's skin.
- Follow the rules of electrical safety when using an electrical appliance.

Preparation

1. Gather supplies
   - Heating pad
   - Towel or flannel cover, if needed
   - Watch   ☐ ☐

Additional Information

8. Ask your supervising nurse for the proper temperature to use to set the heating pad and the length of time for applying it. Remind the person not to change the temperature setting.

Plug in the heating pad and set the thermostat to the proper temperature. Cover the heating pad with a towel or flannel cover, if needed.

2. Focus   ☐ ☐

3. Knock and wait   ☐ ☐

4. Introduce and identify   ☐ ☐

5. Explain   ☐ ☐

6. Place supplies   ☐ ☐

7. Wash hands   ☐ ☐

8. Gather and prepare   ☐ ☐

9. Adjust bed   ☐ ☐

10. Provide privacy   ☐ ☐

Notes:

Procedure

1. Apply the heating pad to the affected area of the person's skin. Adjust the position of the heating pad so that its weight is comfortable for the person. ☐ ☐

2. Make sure the call signal is within the person's reach. ☐ ☐

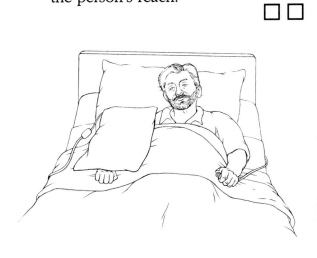

3. Remove the heating pad when the treatment time is up. ☐ ☐

Completion

Additional Information

1. Before you leave, check—
   - Call signal.
   - Body alignment.
   - Bed lowered.
   - Side rails, if used.
   - Comfort.

9. Record—
   - Location of application.
   - Time of application.
   - Duration of application.
   - Person's response to the application.
   Report—
   - Pain.
   - Red or swollen areas.

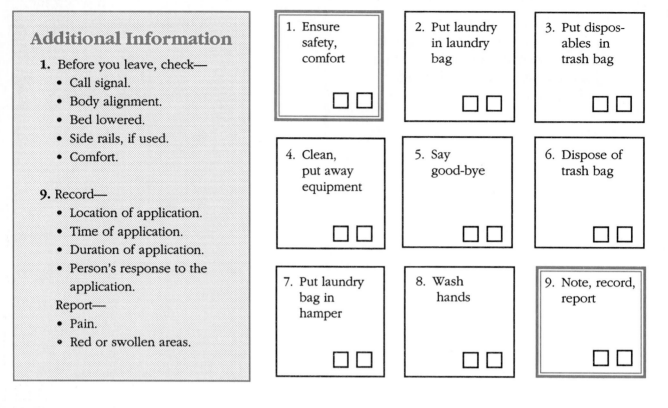

1. Ensure safety, comfort ☐ ☐	2. Put laundry in laundry bag ☐ ☐	3. Put disposables in trash bag ☐ ☐
4. Clean, put away equipment ☐ ☐	5. Say good-bye ☐ ☐	6. Dispose of trash bag ☐ ☐
7. Put laundry bag in hamper ☐ ☐	8. Wash hands ☐ ☐	9. Note, record, report ☐ ☐

_____
Student   Date

_____
Instructor   Date

Skill 66: Applying a Warm Water Bottle

Precautions

- High temperatures can burn a person's skin. Immediately report any signs of burns, pain, redness, or blisters.
- Be especially careful in applying heat to a person who is confused or who has poor sensation in the affected area.

Preparation

1. Gather supplies
   - Warm water bottle
   - Towel or flannel cover for warm water bottle
   - Bath thermometer
   - Watch
   - Paper towels   ☐ ☐

Additional Information

8. Ask your supervising nurse what the proper temperature of the water should be. Fill the bottle 1/2 to 2/3 full with the correct temperature water.
- Check the temperature of the water with the bath thermometer to make sure that it is at the proper temperature.
- Get rid of the air in the bottle by squeezing the bag just until the water level comes up to the top of the bag. Then, without letting go, put the cap on the warm water bottle.
- Dry the bottle with paper towels..
- Turn the bottle upside down to check for leaks.
- Wrap the warm water bottle in a towel or flannel cover.

| 2. Focus ☐ ☐ | 3. Knock and wait ☐ ☐ | 4. Introduce and identify ☐ ☐ |

| 5. Explain ☐ ☐ | 6. Place supplies ☐ ☐ | 7. Wash hands ☐ ☐ |

| 8. Gather and prepare ☐ ☐ | 9. Adjust bed ☐ ☐ | 10. Provide privacy ☐ ☐ |

Notes:

Procedure

1. Apply the wrapped warm water bottle to the prescribed area of the person's skin. Adjust the position of the warm water bottle so that its weight is not uncomfortable to the person. Make sure that the part touching the skin has not become wet.   ☐ ☐

Why? Moist heat burns faster than dry heat.

2. Make sure the call signal is within the person's reach.   ☐ ☐

3. Remove the warm water bottle when the treatment time is up.   ☐ ☐

Completion

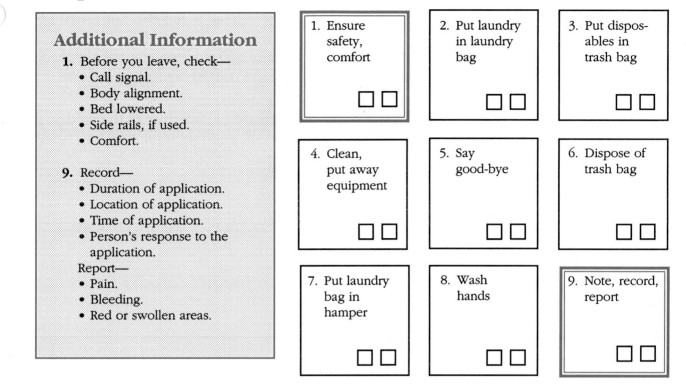

Additional Information

1. Before you leave, check—
   - Call signal.
   - Body alignment.
   - Bed lowered.
   - Side rails, if used.
   - Comfort.

9. Record—
   - Duration of application.
   - Location of application.
   - Time of application.
   - Person's response to the application.
   Report—
   - Pain.
   - Bleeding.
   - Red or swollen areas.

1. Ensure safety, comfort

2. Put laundry in laundry bag

3. Put disposables in trash bag

4. Clean, put away equipment

5. Say good-bye

6. Dispose of trash bag

7. Put laundry bag in hamper

8. Wash hands

9. Note, record, report

_____   _____
Student   Date

_____   _____
Instructor   Date

Completion

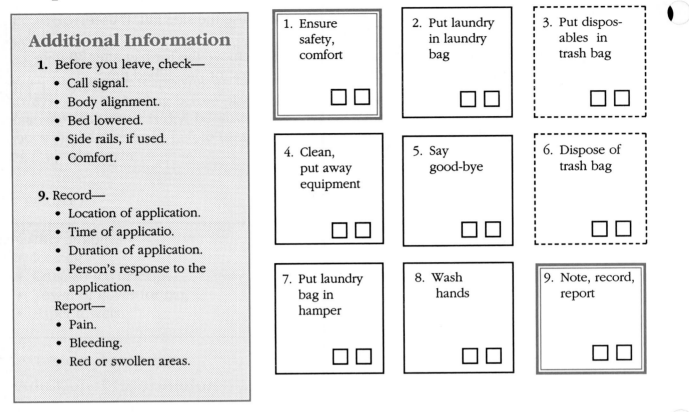

Student _____ Date

Instructor _____ Date

Skill 68: Maintaining Gastric Suctioning

Precautions

- Follow universal precautions and use infection control techniques when handling stomach contents.

Preparation

1. Gather supplies
   - One or two pairs of disposable gloves
   - Lip cream or petroleum jelly and cotton-tipped applicator
   - Plastic trash bag
   - Laundry bag (or plastic bag for wet or soiled linens)
   - Replacement suction container, if needed ☐ ☐

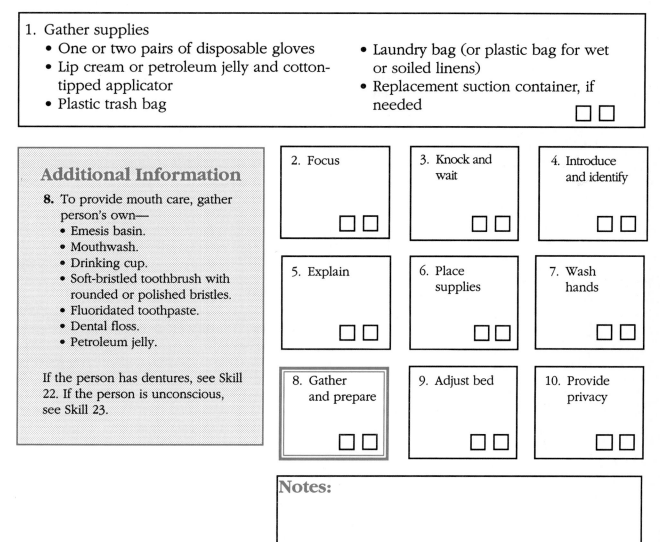

Additional Information

8. To provide mouth care, gather person's own—
   - Emesis basin.
   - Mouthwash.
   - Drinking cup.
   - Soft-bristled toothbrush with rounded or polished bristles.
   - Fluoridated toothpaste.
   - Dental floss.
   - Petroleum jelly.

If the person has dentures, see Skill 22. If the person is unconscious, see Skill 23.

2. Focus ☐ ☐

3. Knock and wait ☐ ☐

4. Introduce and identify ☐ ☐

5. Explain ☐ ☐

6. Place supplies ☐ ☐

7. Wash hands ☐ ☐

8. Gather and prepare ☐ ☐

9. Adjust bed ☐ ☐

10. Provide privacy ☐ ☐

Notes:

1. Provide oral hygiene every 2 hours. ☐ ☐

Why? Most people breathe through the mouth during suctioning, which may cause dryness and irritation.

2. Keep the person's nose clean and apply recommended lubricants to the nasal membranes if cracking, dryness, irritation, or bleeding occurs. (See Skill 59). ☐ ☐

3. Check to make sure the suction is working and that fluid is collecting in the suctioning equipment. ☐ ☐

4. Wear disposable gloves to empty or replace the suctioning equipment as the stomach contents accumulate. Note how much accumulates and its appearance. Report any unusual findings to your supervising nurse. ☐ ☐

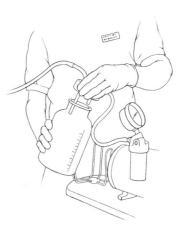

Completion

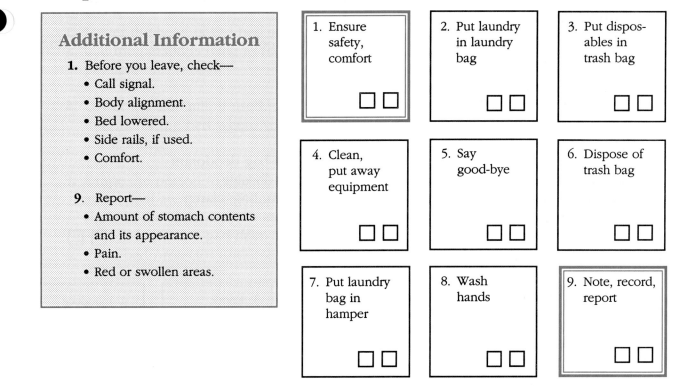

Additional Information

1. Before you leave, check—
- Call signal.
- Body alignment.
- Bed lowered.
- Side rails, if used.
- Comfort.

9. Report—
- Amount of stomach contents and its appearance.
- Pain.
- Red or swollen areas.

---

1. Ensure safety, comfort ☐ ☐

2. Put laundry in laundry bag ☐ ☐

3. Put disposables in trash bag ☐ ☐

4. Clean, put away equipment ☐ ☐

5. Say good-bye ☐ ☐

6. Dispose of trash bag ☐ ☐

7. Put laundry bag in hamper ☐ ☐

8. Wash hands ☐ ☐

9. Note, record, report ☐ ☐

_____

Student   Date

_____

Instructor   Date

Completion

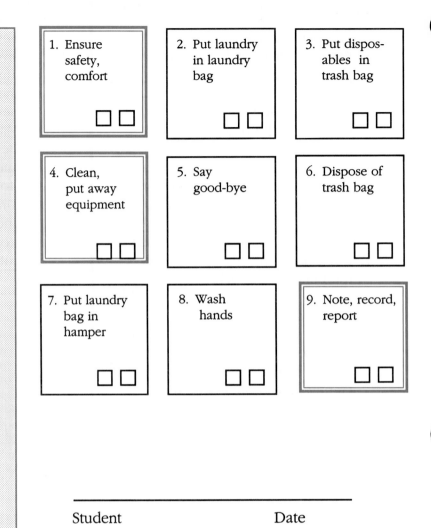

Student   Date

Instructor   Date

Procedure

Remain in
assist the
ed. He or
the person
make the
Common
bent positi
lithotomy
tion. Alway
privacy and
the person
examined.

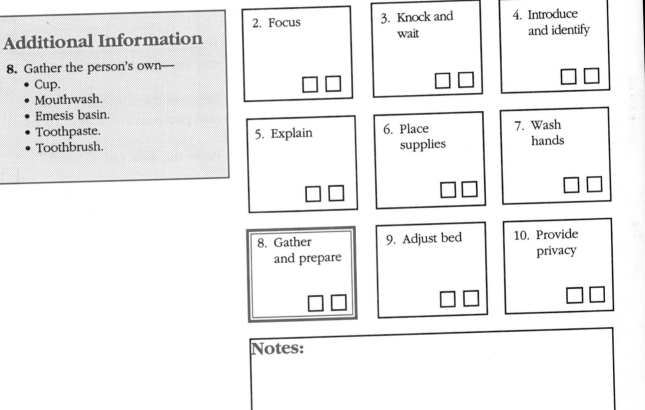

Drapes have bee   ov

view of positions

Skill 70: Collecting Sputum Specimens

Precautions

- Always follow universal precautions and use infection control techniques when collecting sputum.

Preparation

1. Gather supplies.
   - Labeled specimen container
   - Protective eyewear (optional)
   - Disposable gloves
   - Plastic trash bag
   - Towel

   ☐ ☐

Additional Information

8. Gather the person's own—
   - Cup.
   - Mouthwash.
   - Emesis basin.
   - Toothpaste.
   - Toothbrush.

2. Focus ☐ ☐

3. Knock and wait ☐ ☐

4. Introduce and identify ☐ ☐

5. Explain ☐ ☐

6. Place supplies ☐ ☐

7. Wash hands ☐ ☐

8. Gather and prepare ☐ ☐

9. Adjust bed ☐ ☐

10. Provide privacy ☐ ☐

Notes:

Skill 71: Ass[...]

Precautions

- Before the exam[...]
  and what equip[...]

  Note: Your role[...]
  the doctor or nu[...]

Preparation

1. Gather supplies[...]
   - Thermometer
   - Blood pressure c[...]
   - Stethoscope
   - Weight scale
   - Tongue blades
   - Specimen cups la[...]
     name
   - Tape measure
   - Lubricant
   - Alcohol wipes (o[...]
     and alcohol)
   - Cotton-tipped ap[...]

Skill 73: Administering a Vaginal Douche

Precautions

- Follow the physician's order regarding the solution used for the douche.
- Warm the solution to provide comfort to the woman.
- Do not administer a douche during a woman's menstruation.
- Always ask the woman to urinate before administering the douche.

Preparation

1. Gather supplies
   - IV pole
   - Douche solution or commercially prepared douche
   - Irrigation equipment
   - Disposable bed protector
   - Bath blanket or sheet
   - Disposable gloves
   - Plastic trash bag
   - Laundry bag (or plastic bag for wet or soiled linens)
   - Two washcloths
   - Towel
   ☐ ☐

Additional Information

8. Gather the woman's own—
   - Washbasin.
   - Bedpan.
   - Powder.

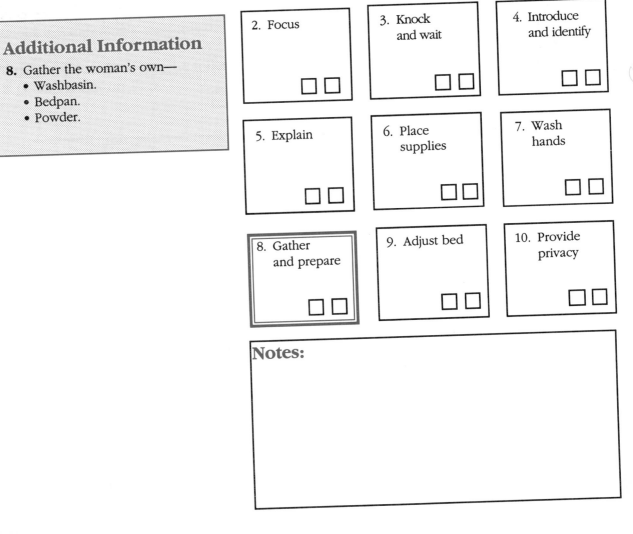

2. Focus ☐ ☐

3. Knock and wait ☐ ☐

4. Introduce and identify ☐ ☐

5. Explain ☐ ☐

6. Place supplies ☐ ☐

7. Wash hands ☐ ☐

8. Gather and prepare ☐ ☐

9. Adjust bed ☐ ☐

10. Provide privacy ☐ ☐

Notes:

Procedure

1. Warm the prescribed solution by running the container of solution under warm water or placing it in a basin of warm water. Hook the irrigation equipment to an IV pole. If using a commercially prepared douche, follow the manufacturer's directions. ☐ ☐

2. Lower the head of the bed so that it is flat (or as low as the woman can tolerate). ☐ ☐

3. Lower the side rail, if used, on the side where you are working. ☐ ☐

4. Help the woman into a supine position. ☐ ☐

5. Put a disposable bed protector under her buttocks to protect the bedding. ☐ ☐

6. Drape her perineal area with a bath blanket. ☐ ☐

7. Elevate the woman's pelvis by helping her onto a powdered bed pan. ☐ ☐

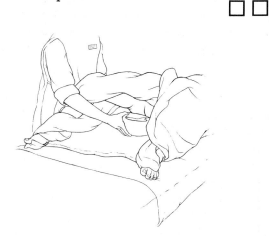

8. Put on disposable gloves. ☐ ☐

9. Separate the woman's labia and place the nozzle of the prepared douche into her vagina. Direct the nozzle downward and backward and gently rotate it within her vagina while you are inserting it. Insert it 3 to 4 inches. If using a commercially prepared douche, follow the manufacturer's directions. ☐ ☐

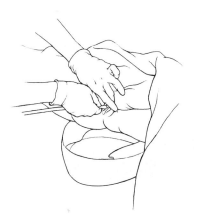

10. Slowly squeeze the prepared douche so that the solution flows into the woman's vagina, or allow the solution to flow from the irrigation container. When all the solution is gone, remove the nozzle. Throw away the disposable douche container into the plastic trash bag. ☐ ☐

11. If possible, help the woman into a semi-Fowler's or sitting position. ☐ ☐

12. Allow the solution to cleanse her vagina and run out into the bed pan. ☐ ☐

13. Provide any perineal care, if necessary. ☐ ☐

14. Dry the woman's skin and labia with a clean towel. ☐ ☐

15. Remove the bedpan.

16. Remove the disposable gloves and discard them in a plastic trash bag. ☐ ☐

17. Raise the side rail, if used. ☐ ☐

18. Adjust the head of the bed. ☐ ☐

Completion

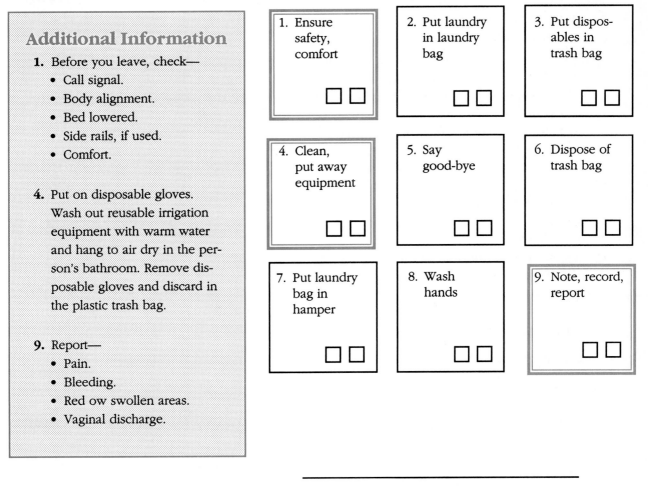

1. Ensure safety, comfort ☐ ☐

2. Put laundry in laundry bag ☐ ☐

3. Put disposables in trash bag ☐ ☐

4. Clean, put away equipment ☐ ☐

5. Say good-bye ☐ ☐

6. Dispose of trash bag ☐ ☐

7. Put laundry bag in hamper ☐ ☐

8. Wash hands ☐ ☐

9. Note, record, report ☐ ☐

_____

Student   Date

_____

Instructor   Date

Skill 74: Assisting with a Whirlpool Bath

Precautions

- During a whirlpool bath, the increased blood flow to some parts of a person's body might cause him to become dizzy or faint. Observe the person often for signs of faintness, dizziness, fatigue, or weakness.
- Make sure the water temperature is between 95 and 110 degrees Fahrenheit to prevent burns or injury.
- Never leave the person alone in the tub.

Preparation

1. Gather supplies
   - One towel
   - Laundry bag (or plastic bag for wet or soiled linens)
   - Bath thermometer ☐ ☐

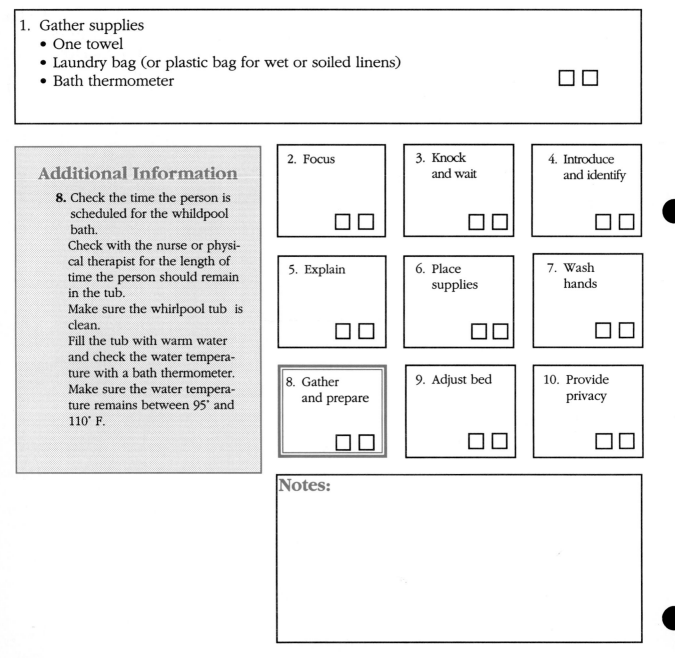

Additional Information

8. Check the time the person is scheduled for the whildpool bath.
Check with the nurse or physical therapist for the length of time the person should remain in the tub.
Make sure the whirlpool tub is clean.
Fill the tub with warm water and check the water temperature with a bath thermometer.
Make sure the water temperature remains between 95° and 110° F.

2. Focus ☐ ☐

3. Knock and wait ☐ ☐

4. Introduce and identify ☐ ☐

5. Explain ☐ ☐

6. Place supplies ☐ ☐

7. Wash hands ☐ ☐

8. Gather and prepare ☐ ☐

9. Adjust bed ☐ ☐

10. Provide privacy ☐ ☐

Notes:

Procedure

1. Place a chair near the whirlpool. ☐ ☐

2. Help the person remove his clothing. Help him into the tub. ☐ ☐

3. On the whirlpool control, press the turbine (agitation or mixing) button and adjust for desired turbulence (motion). ☐ ☐

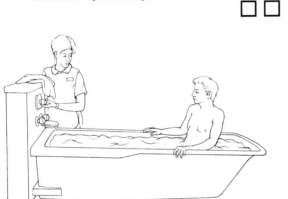

4. Observe the person often for signs of faintness, dizziness, fatigue, or weakness. ☐ ☐

Note: If the person becomes faint or dizzy, let the water out of the tub and lower the person's head forward. Call for help by using the emergency call button beside the tub.

5. Remain with the person until the bath is finished. ☐ ☐

6. Help the person out of the tub and help, as needed, with toweling dry and dressing. ☐ ☐

Completion

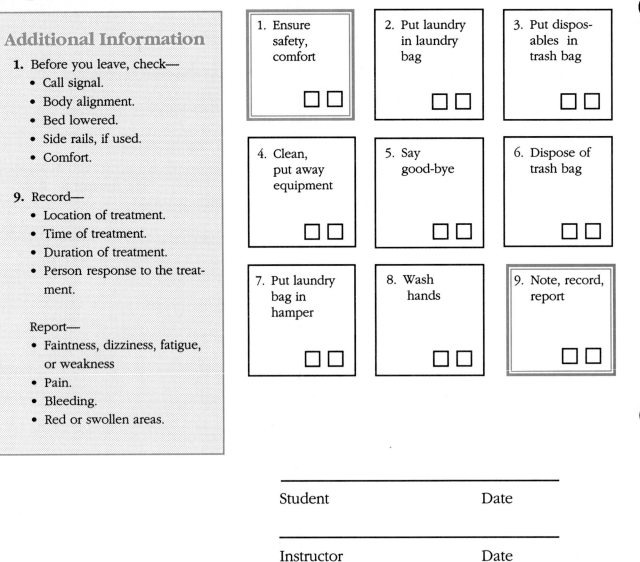

Additional Information

1. Before you leave, check—
   - Call signal.
   - Body alignment.
   - Bed lowered.
   - Side rails, if used.
   - Comfort.

9. Record—
   - Location of treatment.
   - Time of treatment.
   - Duration of treatment.
   - Person response to the treatment.

   Report—
   - Faintness, dizziness, fatigue, or weakness
   - Pain.
   - Bleeding.
   - Red or swollen areas.

1. Ensure safety, comfort ☐ ☐

2. Put laundry in laundry bag ☐ ☐

3. Put disposables in trash bag ☐ ☐

4. Clean, put away equipment ☐ ☐

5. Say good-bye ☐ ☐

6. Dispose of trash bag ☐ ☐

7. Put laundry bag in hamper ☐ ☐

8. Wash hands ☐ ☐

9. Note, record, report ☐ ☐

_____
Student   Date

_____
Instructor   Date

Appendix

Raising and Lowering Side Rails Unit 6, Section 2, Activity 3

Precautions

- When using side rails, make sure they are in the locked position once they are raised or lowered.

- If the rail will not lock properly, stay with the person and call someone to fix the rail.

Procedure

1. Lift the side rail and raise it to its locked position.

2. Unlock the side rail.

3. Lower the side rail to its original position.

Using Brakes on Beds, Wheelchairs, and Shower Chairs

Precautions

- Always be sure that the lock is secure on the brake and the person's feet are on the footrests.

- If the brakes are not working properly, report this observation to your supervising nurse.

Procedure

1. Find the brakes on the bed.

2. Move the brakes on the bed to their locked position.

3. Release the brakes on the bed.

4. Find the brakes, footrests and other safety features on the wheelchair and shower chair.

5. Move the brakes on the wheelchair and shower chair to their locked positions.

6. Release the brakes on the wheelchair and shower chair.

Student Worksheet 2

Demonstration: First Aid for Falls Unit 6, Section 4, Activity 3

Precautions

- When helping a person walk or move, clear obstacles out of the way. Remember, prevention is the best safety measure.

- If the person falls, do not leave him.

- If the person falls, do not move him.

Procedure: When a Person is Falling

1. If possible, catch the person. You should keep your feet apart, back straight, and knees slightly bent.

2. Put your arms around the person's waist or underarms, keep him close to your body, and lower him slowly to floor by sliding him down your leg.

3. Call for help.

4. Help the person to be comfortable.
   Reassure him
   Do not leave him
   Do not move the person until he has been checked by your supervising nurse and she instructs you to do so.

Completion

1. When your supervising nurse directs you, help move the person.
   Make him comfortable and put the call signal within his reach.

3. Wash your hands.

4. Give necessary information to your supervising nurse, to make sure the person is all right and to offer reassurance.

5. Check the person, as directed by your supervising nurse, to make sure the person is all right and to offer reassurance.

Procedure: When a Person Has Fallen

1. Look around. (Survey the scene)

2. Look at the person.
   Does the person respond?
   Is the person breathing?

3. Call for help.

4. If the person is responsive, ask him what happened.
   Is there any pain?
   Check his vital signs, as directed by your supervising nurse.
   Help your supervising nurse as she does a head-to-toe exam.

5. Help the person to be comfortable.
   Reassure him
   Do not leave him
   Do not move him until he has been checked by the supervising physcian, or EMS personnel, and has directed you to move him

Completion

1. When your supervising nurse, the physician, or EMS personnel direct you, help move the person.

2. Make him comfortable and put the call signal within his reach.

3. Wash your hands.

4. Provide necessary information to your supervising nurse for the incident report.

5. Check the person, as directed by your supervising nurse, to make sure the person is all right and to offer reassurance.

Student Worksheet 3
Activities of Daily Living (ADL) Flow Sheet

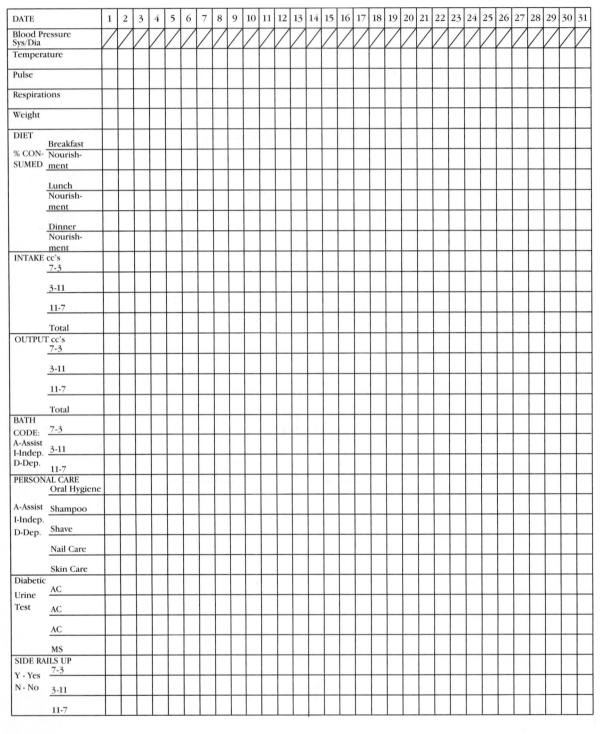

DATE		1	2	3	4	5	6	7	8	9	10	11	12	13	14	15	16	17	18	19	20	21	22	23	24	25	26	27	28	29	30	31
Blood Pressure Sys/Dia																																
Temperature																																
Pulse																																
Respirations																																
Weight																																
DIET % CON-SUMED	Breakfast Nourish-ment																															
	Lunch Nourish-ment																															
	Dinner Nourish-ment																															
INTAKE cc's	7-3																															
	3-11																															
	11-7																															
	Total																															
OUTPUT cc's	7-3																															
	3-11																															
	11-7																															
	Total																															
BATH CODE: A-Assist I-Indep. D-Dep.	7-3																															
	3-11																															
	11-7																															
PERSONAL CARE A-Assist I-Indep. D-Dep.	Oral Hygiene																															
	Shampoo																															
	Shave																															
	Nail Care																															
	Skin Care																															
Diabetic Urine Test	AC																															
	AC																															
	AC																															
	MS																															
SIDE RAILS UP Y - Yes N - No	7-3																															
	3-11																															
	11-7																															

LAST NAME	FIRST NAME	INITIAL	ATTENDING PHYSICIAN	ROOM NO.	PATIENT NO.

ACTIVITIES OF DAILY LIVING FLOW SHEET

DATE		1	2	3	4	5	6	7	8	9	10	11	12	13	14	15	16	17	18	19	20	21	22	23	24	25	26	27	28	29	30	31
UP IN CHAIR	7-3																															
A-Assist	3-11																															
I-Indep.																																
D-Dep.	11-7																															
ROM EXERCISES	7-3																															
A-Active																																
P-Passive	3-11																															
POSITION CHANGED	7-3																															
A-Assist	3-11																															
I-Indep.																																
D-Dep.	11-7																															
BLADDER ACTION	7-3																															
C-Continent	3-11																															
I-Incontinent																																
Foley 0 × 0	11-7																															
BOWEL ACTION	7-3																															
C-Continent	3-11																															
I-Incontinent																																
0 × 0	11-7																															
CONSISTENCY	7-3																															
L-Liquid	3-11																															
S-Soft formed																																
H-Hard formed	11-7																															
PERI CARE	7-3																															
A-Assist	3-11																															
I-Indep.																																
D-Dep.	11-7																															
OTHER																																
Nurse Assistant Initials	A.M.																															
	P.M.																															
	NOC.																															

Nurse Assistant Signature and Initials: _____

LAST NAME	FIRST NAME	INITIAL	ATTENDING PHYSICIAN	ROOM NO.	PATIENT NO.

Student Worksheet 4

Before and After Menu Unit 12, Section 1, Activity 1

	Before	Foods Group Serving	After
Breakfast	1 Banana 1 egg cereal	Grain Vegetables Fruit Meat Milk Fat	
Mid-Morning Snack	1 apple Coke	Grain Vegetables Fruit Meat Milk Fat	
Lunch	1 Coke	Grain Vegetables Fruit Meat Milk Fat	
Mid-Afternoon Snack	Veggie Salad Hot dog orange juice	Grain Vegetables Fruit Meat Milk Fat Grain	
Dinner Evening Snack	Rice Broiled chicken Water	Vegetables Fruit Meat Milk Fat	
Total		Grain Vegetables Fruit Meat Milk Fat	

From Ounces to cc's

1 oz. = 30 cc

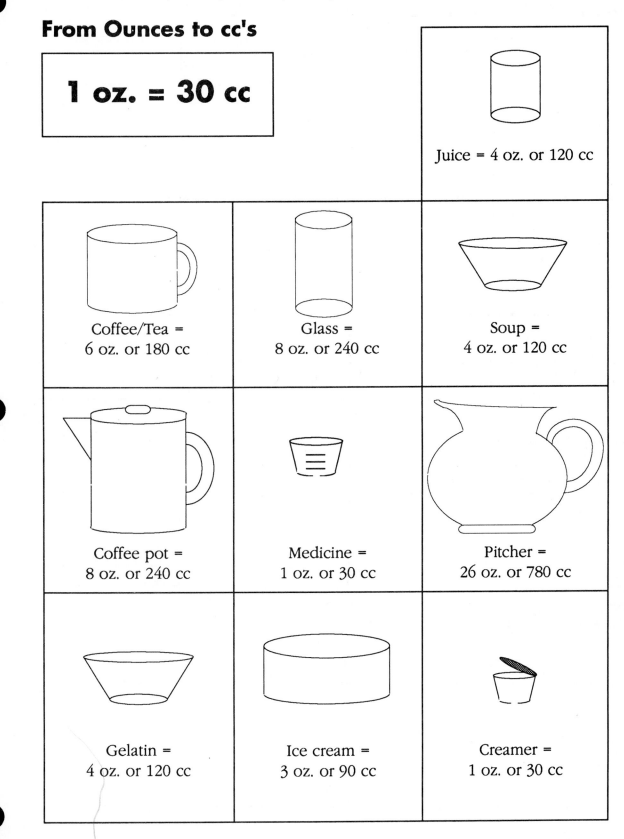

Juice = 4 oz. or 120 cc

Coffee/Tea =
6 oz. or 180 cc

Glass =
8 oz. or 240 cc

Soup =
4 oz. or 120 cc

Coffee pot =
8 oz. or 240 cc

Medicine =
1 oz. or 30 cc

Pitcher =
26 oz. or 780 cc

Gelatin =
4 oz. or 120 cc

Ice cream =
3 oz. or 90 cc

Creamer =
1 oz. or 30 cc

Student Worksheet 6

Intake Form Unit 12, Section 3, Activity 1

Meal	Time	Food Served	Description	Amount Eaten
Breakfast				
Mid-Morning Snack				
Lunch				
Mid-Afternoon Snack				
Dinner				
Evening Snack				
Last Name	First Name, Initial	Attending Physician	Room No.	Patient No.